CATEGORY: GENERAL PRACTI

DRS BRAY, SMITH, PATEL
TANNA & WHITER
St. Andrews Medical Practice
50 Oakleigh Road North
Whetstone London N20 9EX
Tel: 020 8445 0475

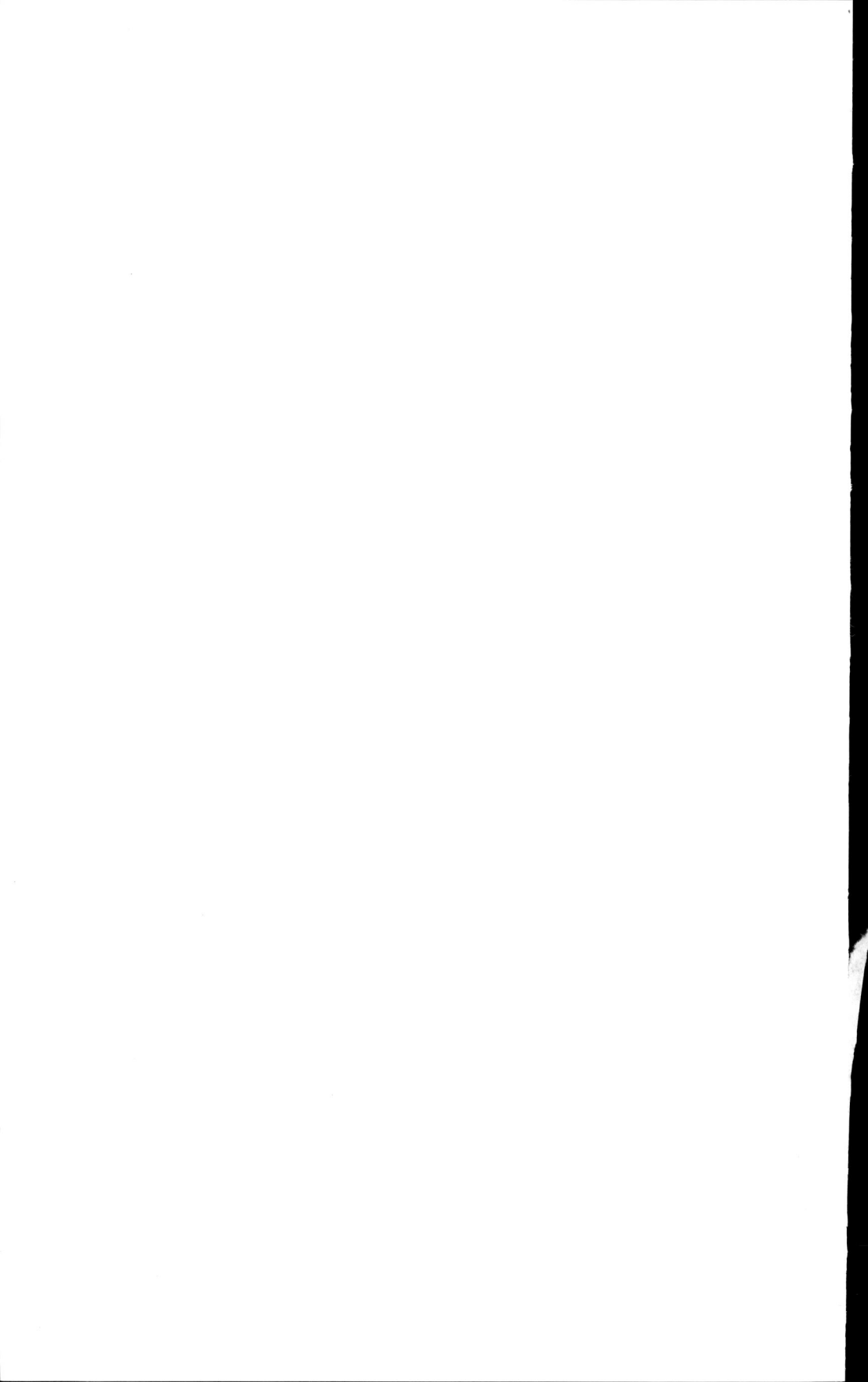

DECISION-MAKING IN GENERAL PRACTICE

DECISION-MAKING IN GENERAL PRACTICE

Edited by

Michael Sheldon
Department of Community Health
Queens Medical Centre
Nottingham

John Brooke
Digital Equipment Co Ltd
Reading

and

Alan Rector
Medical Computation Unit
Manchester Royal Infirmary

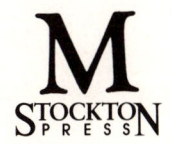

M
STOCKTON PRESS

© The Contributors 1985

All rights reserved. No reproduction, copy or transmission
of this publication may be made without written permission.

No paragraph of this publication may be reproduced, copied
or transmitted save with written permission or in accordance
with the provisions of the Copyright Act 1956 (as amended).

Any person who does any unauthorised act in relation to
this publication may be liable to criminal prosecution and
civil claims for damages.

First published 1985

Published in the United Kingdom by
THE MACMILLAN PRESS LTD
Houndmills, Basingstoke, Hampshire RG21 2XS
and London
Companies and representatives
throughout the world

Printed in Great Britain by
Camelot Press Ltd,
Southampton

British Library Cataloguing in Publication Data
Decision-making in general practice.
1. Medicine, Clinical — Decision making
I. Sheldon, Michael G. II. Brooke, John
III. Rector, Alan
616'.001'9 RC48
ISBN 0-333-36626-3

Published in the United States and Canada by
Stockton Press
15 East 26th Street, New York, NY 10010

Library of Congress Cataloguing in Publication Data
Main entry under title:
Decision-making in general practice.
Based on a conference held at Holme Pierrepont,
Nottingham, England, in Dec. 1983.
1. Family medicine–Decision making–Congresses.
2. Medicine–Decision making–Congresses. I. Sheldon,
Michael, 1941- . II. Brooke, John, 1951- .
III. Rector, Alan. [DNLM: 1. Decision Making–
Congresses. 2. Family Practice–Congresses.
W 89 D294 1983]
R729.5.G4D43 1985   610   85-8915
ISBN 0-943818-11-7

Contents

Workshop Participants	vii
Preface	xiii
Acknowledgements	xv

1. The Consultation: A Multi-purpose Framework *John G.R. Howie* 1
2. The Consultation Process *Frank Martin Hull* 13
3. Discussion of the Papers by Howie and Hull *Ann Cartwright* 27
4. Patient-centred and Doctor-centred Models of Clinical Decision-making *Ian R. McWhinney* 31
5. A Model for the General Practice Consultation *Joseph H. Levenstein* 47
6. Discussion of the Papers by McWhinney and Levenstein *David Pendleton* 55
7. Diagnosis: Process not Product *Janet Gale and Philip Marsden* 59
8. Discussion of the Paper by Gale and Marsden *Frank Martin Hull* 91
9. Clinical Decision = Patient with Problem + Doctor with Problem *John B. Brooke and Michael G. Sheldon* 95
10. Knowledge and Judgement in Decision-making *John Fox* 108
11. Implications of Research on Clinical Decision-making for the Design of Decision Support Systems *Alan L. Rector and David C. Dodson* 119
12. Factors Influencing Referrals by General Practitioners to Consultants *Bernard J. M. Aulbers* 131
13. A Discussion on Aids to Decision-making in the Consultation *Mike Fitter* 141
14. Developing a Unitary Model of the Clinical Management Process *Thomas R. Taylor and Michael J. Gordon* 145
15. The Probabilistic Paradigm as the Basic Science of the Practice of Family Medicine *Richard I. Feinbloom* 161
16. Discussion of the Papers by Taylor and Feinbloom *Benjamin J. Essex* 167
17. The Surface Anatomy of Primary Health Care — Does Consultation Analysis Contribute? *Nigel C. H. Stott* 169
18. Decision Analysis in General Practice *Benjamin J. Essex* 183
19. Discussion of the Papers by Stott and Essex *Mike A. Pringle* 199

20. A Computer-assisted Diagnostic Decision System for Dyspepsia *Robin P. Knill-Jones, William M. Dunwoodie and Gerard P. Crean*	203
21. The Health Problem and Tools for the Computer *Bent G. Bentsen*	221
22. The Paper Patient — A Device for Investigation into General Practice *J. Ridderikhoff*	239
23. Discussion of the Papers by Bentsen and Ridderikhoff *Paul Keith Hodgkin*	255
24. Overview and Implications for Medical Education *George A. Brown*	257

Workshop Participants

Bernard J.M. AULBERS
  General Practitioner and
    Senior Lecturer in the
  Department of General Practice at the
  Erasmus University of Rotterdam
  Mathenesserlaan 264A
  3021 HR Rotterdam
  The Netherlands

Bent Guttorm BENTSEN
  Department of Community Medicine
  University of Trondheim
  Regional Hospital
  Park Building
  7000 Trondheim
  Norway

Michael J. BOLAND
  General Practice Tutor to the
    West Cork Pilot Study
  Lurriga
  Skibbereen
  Co Cork
  Ireland

John B. BROOKE
  Human Factors Specialist
  European Engineering
  Digital Equipment Co Ltd
  PO Box 121
  Reading
  Berkshire
  UK

George A. BROWN
  Reader in University Teaching Methods
  School of Education
  University of Nottingham
  University Park
  Nottingham
  UK

Kenneth BURCH
  General Practitioner
  The Health Centre
  East Street
  Thame
  Oxon
  UK

Ann CARTWRIGHT
  Director of the
    Institute for Social Studies in Medical
    Care
  14 South Hill Park
  London NW3
  UK

Gerard P. CREAN*
  Director of the Diagnostic
    Methodology Research Unit
  Southern General Hospital
  Glasgow G51 4TF
  UK

* A co-contributor who did not attend the Workshop.

Workshop Participants

Donald L. CROMBIE
  General Practitioner and
    Director of the Research Unit of
    the RCGP
  Lordswood House
  54 Lordswood Road
  Harborne
  Birmingham B17 9DB
  UK

David C. DODSON
  Department of Community Health
  University of Nottingham
  Queen's Medical Centre
  Nottingham NG7 2UH
  UK

  Present address:
  Department of Computer Sciences
  City University
  Northampton Square
  London EC1V 0HB

William M. DUNWOODIE
  Department of General Practice
  University of Glasgow
  Woodside Health Centre
  Barr Street
  Glasgow
  UK

J. Mark ELWOOD
  Professor and Head of Department
    of Community Health
  Queen's Medical Centre
  Clifton Boulevard
  Nottingham NG7 2UH
  UK

Benjamin J. ESSEX
  General Practitioner and Consultant
    to the World Health Organization
  3 Alleyn Road
  London SE1 8AB
  UK

Richard I. FEINBLOOM
  Clinical Associate Professor
  Department of Family Medicine
  State University of New York
  Stony Brook
  New York 11733
  USA

Mike FITTER
  Senior Research Officer
  MRC/SSRC Social and Applied
    Psychology Unit
  University of Sheffield
  Sheffield S10 2TN
  UK

Richard FITTON
  General Practitioner
  West Gorton Medical Centre
  6A Wenlock Way
  Manchester M12 5LH
  UK

John FOX
  Head of Biomedical Computing Unit
  Imperial Cancer Research Fund
  Lincoln's Inn Fields
  London WC2A 3PX
  UK

Paul FREELING
  Reader and Head of Sub-Department
    of General Practice
  St George's Hospital Medical School
  Cranmer Terrace
  Tooting
  London SW17 0RE
  UK

Workshop Participants

Janet GALE
  Lecturer in Educational Technology
  Institute of Educational Technology
  Open University
  Walton Hall
  Milton Keynes MK7 6AA
  UK

Michael J. GORDON
  Associate Professor
  Clinical Management Research Group
  Department of Family Medicine
  University of Washington
  Seattle
  Washington 98195
  USA

Paul Keith HODGKIN
  Lecturer in General Practice
  Department of General Practice
  Rusholme Health Centre
  Manchester M13
  UK

John G.R. HOWIE
  Professor of General Practice
  University of Edinburgh
  20 West Richmond Street
  Edinburgh EH8 9DX
  UK

Frank Martin HULL
  Senior Lecturer in General Practice
  Department of General Practice
  Medical School
  University of Birmingham
  Edgbaston
  Birmingham B15 2TJ
  UK

Robin P. KNILL-JONES
  Diagnostic Methodology Research Unit
  Southern General Hospital
  Glasgow G51 4TF
  UK

Robert V.H. JONES
  General Practitioner and
    Senior Lecturer in the Department of
    General Practice of Exeter University
  Foxenholts
  Covehill Lane
  Seaton
  Devon
  UK

Joseph H. LEVENSTEIN
  South African Academy of Family
    Practice/Primary Care
  Rooms 24/25, Medical House
  Central Square
  Pinelands 7430
  Cape Town
  South Africa

Ian R. McWHINNEY
  Professor and Chairman of the
    Department of Family Medicine
  Kresge Building
  The University of Western Ontario
  London
  Ontario N6A 5C1
  Canada

Philip MARSDEN
  Consultant Physician and Clinical Tutor
  Postgraduate Medical Centre
  Greenwich District Hospital
  Van Brugh Hill
  London SE10
  UK

Workshop Participants

Walter MROZINZKI
Medical Computation Unit
University of Manchester
Manchester Royal Infirmary
Oxford Road
Manchester M13 9WL
UK

David PENDLETON
Fellow in Managerial Psychology
The King's Fund College
2 Palace Court
London W2 4HS
UK

Ian PRIBAN
British Consortium for Innovation
27 Bedford Square
London WC1B 3HW
UK

Mike A. PRINGLE
General Practitioner and
 Part-time Clinical Lecturer in
 General Practice
The Health Centre
High Street
Collingham
Newark
Nottinghamshire
UK

Alan L. RECTOR
Senior Lecturer in Computational
 Methods in Medical Science
Medical Computation Unit
University of Manchester
Manchester Royal Infirmary
Oxford Road
Manchester M13 9WL
UK

Bernard B. REISS
Director of Studies in General Practice
University of Cambridge School of
 Clinical Medicine
The Clinical School
Addenbrooke's Hospital
Hills Road
Cambridge CB2 2QQ
UK

J. RIDDERIKHOFF
Senior Lecturer in Family Medicine
Erasmus University of Rotterdam
PO Box 1738
3000 DR Rotterdam
The Netherlands

Michael G. SHELDON
Senior Lecturer in General Practice
Department of Community Health
University of Nottingham Medical
 School
Queen's Medical Centre
Clifton Boulevard
Nottingham NG7 2UH
UK

John Llewelyn SKINNER
General Practitioner and
 Part-time Lecturer in General Practice
Waterloo Lane
Trowell
Nottinghamshire NG9 3QQ
UK

J.A. SMAL
Psychologist
Research and Development
Department of Medical Education
State University of Utrecht
Bijlhouwerstraat 6
3511 ZC Utrecht
The Netherlands

Workshop Participants

C. Michael SPENCER
  General Practitioner and
    Clinical Tutor in General Practice
  at the University of Nottingham
  Oxford House Medical Centre
  Easthorpe Street
  Ruddington
  Nottingham
  UK

David John SPIEGELHALTER
  Statistician
  MRC Biostatistics Unit
  MRC Centre
  Hills Road
  Cambridge CB2 2QH
  UK

Ian M. STANLEY
  Division of General Practice
  Clinical Sciences Building
  St James's Hospital
  Leeds
  LS9 7TF
  UK

Norman STODDART
  General Practitioner
  The Surgery
  St Wilfrid's Square
  Calverton
  Nottingham
  UK

Nigel C.H. STOTT
  Senior Lecturer
  Department of General Practice
  Welsh National School of Medicine
  Heath Park
  Cardiff
  UK

Ian G. TAIT
  General Practitioner and
    Course Organiser
  The Surgery
  15 Lee Road
  Aldeburgh
  Suffolk
  UK

Timothy TAULKE-JOHNSON
  General Practitioner
  129 Red Lion Road
  Tolworth
  Surrey KT6 7QY
  UK

Thomas R. TAYLOR
  Associate Professor
  Department of Family Medicine
  Research Section JD-13
  University of Washington
  Seattle
  Washington 98195
  USA

F. TOUW-OTTEN
  Senior Lecturer and Head of Research
    Section
  Department of General Practice
  University of Utrecht
  Mariahoek 6
  3511 LD Utrecht
  The Netherlands

Roger L. WARD
  Medical Sciences Liaison Division
  Upjohn Ltd
  Fleming Way
  Crawley
  West Sussex RH10 2NJ
  UK

David Gregor WILKINSON
  Research Worker and Hon. Senior
    Registrar
  General Practice Research Unit
  Institute of Psychiatry
  De Crespigny Park
  Denmark Hill
  London SE5 8AF
  UK

John WRIGHT
  Head of Division of General Practice
  Clinical Sciences Building
  St James's Hospital
  Beckett Street
  Leeds LS9 7TF
  UK

Luke ZANDER
  Senior Lecturer
  Department of General Practice
  St Thomas's Hospital
  50 Kennington Road
  London SE11
  UK

Preface

This book contains the collected papers and ensuing discussions at a conference entitled *Decision-making in General Practice* held at Holme Pierrepont, Nottingham, England in December 1983.

The stimulation for this workshop lay in a research project at the Department of Community Health at the University of Nottingham. This project, funded by the Medical Research Council, was aimed at producing computer-based decision support systems for general practitioners. As part of the ground-work, we undertook a review of the literature relating to decision-making in general practice, and were surprised how little there was. There were many papers on the topic of medical decision-making in general, but few of the reported studies had tackled the problems of general practice, and there was no central core of journals or books that we could turn to to locate further information. Furthermore, the material that we did find tended to be spread over a number of years, and the same names kept cropping up over and over again.

It was obvious to us that while there were other people working in the same area of research, there were only limited opportunities for communication between them. A forum at which all could discuss this topic of common interest seemed to be an important requirement for the progression of research. We therefore made some tentative enquiries of all the people whose names we had come across, and much to our surprise the great majority of them agreed to come to the workshop.

This book contains the contributions made to the workshop by the invited speakers, and also attempts to summarise the discussion of the papers. A wide range of disciplines and points of view were represented. There were medical practitioners, social scientists, psychologists, computer scientists, medical educationalists and general practitioners. The delegates to the workshop came from many countries, including the Netherlands, Norway, the USA, Canada, South Africa and the UK.

Because of this wide range of backgrounds, the reader may detect disagreements between various authors represented in this book and in the summaries of the discussion. We do not intend to try and resolve any of these disagreements. We feel that to do so would be to disguise the current state of the art in this area of research and enquiry. On the contrary, we hope that the juxtaposition of these differing points of view will provide further food for thought and will stimulate more research in this area.

M.G.S.
J.B.
A.L.R.

Acknowledgements

The workshop owes a great deal of its success to Alison Langham, who, despite the scattering of the Nottingham research group to various corners of the country, managed to hold everything together whilst doing all the many tasks that administration of a project of this kind requires, in particular the irksome ones of chasing contributors, producing material for precirculation, and keeping the other members of the research team in order.

We also thank Joyce Gilbert, Sheila Kelsey and Judy Rose for the care, tolerance and patience required to turn the conference proceedings into a book. Any mistakes in this book are the fault of the editors and not the secretaries.

We gratefully acknowledge financial help for the conference from:

The Department of Community Health, Nottingham University;
Medical Sciences Liaison (MSL) Division of Upjohn Ltd;
ICI Pharmaceuticals;
The King's Fund.

1
The Consultation: A Multi-purpose Framework

John G.R. Howie

It is difficult to trace the exact origins of the contemporary interest in clinical decision-making. It is now more than a decade since a group of Glasgow physicians (Taylor et al., 1971) analysed how their colleagues used clinical and laboratory information to diagnose and manage thyroid illness. At about the same time, a multi-disciplinary team developed a mathematical model which revolutionised the accuracy of pre-operative differentiation between adrenal hyperplasia and Conn's syndrome (Aitchison et al., 1971). The rapid development of computer technology was used to experiment in many other fields, the work of de Dombal (1971 a & b) in the field of management of abdominal pain reflecting the potential, the interest and the difficulties of the field. In 1967, Feinstein produced his classic monograph on 'Clinical Judgement' which drew attention to some of the differences between the way doctors are taught to practise medicine and actually carry out their clinical work.

The coincidence of events like these with the desire to define the discipline of general practice has been both fortuitous and natural. General practice is governed by the same principles as is the practice of medicine in hospital but, because its context is so different, it needs and uses a substantially different base of knowledge and set of skills. Inevitably, the study of decision-making in general practice has attracted academic attention. Using the word 'academic' in its better meaning, this involves the careful analysis of the clinical behaviour of doctors. Only after a sound analysis of what doctors do, can teaching and practice be based on a synthesis from first principles rather than on a chance adaptation of policies based on so-called 'experience'. At the other end of the scale, the word 'academic' also implies irrelevance. The temptations for university clinical staff, educationists and psychologists to construct unwieldy flow diagrams of behaviour or to milk unsafe numerical data far past the bounds of commonsense have to be resisted steadfastly.

This chapter attempts to describe a simple framework for analysing or synthesising what happens at any interaction between a patient and a doctor. It is presented at a simple level - perhaps even a simplistic level - to identify and use the few fundamental principles which are common to all meetings between all doctors and all patients anywhere. From there it can be used as a basis to build whatever more advanced structure the clinician, the teacher, the researcher, the auditor or the planner may need for his own purposes at any one time. The model* must be compatible with observed and measured reality or it has no basis in science; it must be sensibly flexible or it loses the sensitivity required of an art.

The first part of the chapter identifies some of the historical reasons which have contributed to the need to have a framework for thinking about what happens at a consultation. The second part of the chapter presents the framework itself. The third part of the chapter attempts to defend the validity of the framework in the context of the commonest (although not most complex) single area of general practice work, and concludes by referring briefly to some of the uses to which it may be put.

BACKGROUND

Time and Beliefs

A patient having a myocardial infarction in 1955 would have spent six weeks lying in bed with one pillow as the only concession to the outside world. In 1965, the same patient would have received heparin six-hourly, been started on oral anticoagulants and had to learn to adapt to a life punctuated by pill-taking, blood-letting and the do's and dont's implicit in the customs of the decade. By 1975, coronary care ambulances and units had become the new fashion, although the contrasting potential benefits of home care and early mobilisation were attracting serious attention.

Senility was a common 'cause' of death at the start of the twentieth century - but custom has seen the term lapse. Was the peak of asthma 'deaths' in the 1960s only due to over-use of inhalers or was it contributed to by a new awareness of the large number of patients who have problems with breathing difficulties? Is non-accidental injury a new problem or a new name for a centuries-old reality?

The rate at which 'facts' become obsolete is known to be high and increasing. Most doctors with any insight into their craft will think carefully before equating the present views of 'truth' with 'right' as against 'wrong'. The first essential of a model or framework is that

---

* Professor Howie has suggested that the word 'framework' may be more appropriate. We have left the original term 'model' in this paper as the discussion would otherwise be apparently unrelated. As is apparent from the following paragraph, Professor Howie uses the terms 'framework' and model interchangeably.

it should be able to accommodate the fashions and beliefs of the times and recognise that appropriate care for patients may have to be placed not only in the setting of current beliefs but also against the backdrop of those that were held once - or may come to be held in the future!

Needs and Expectations

No-one disputes the importance of dealing with patients as individuals within the context of their own culture and environment. Expectations are derived from past experience of health and illness both at a personal level and as observed in relatives, neighbours, friends and colleagues. They are influenced by public and professional attitudes and by the media, and by the services offered by local doctors both in hospital and in general practice.

Appropriate care depends on the background, insight and personality of the patient. One patient will be reassured by no more than the word of the general practitioner, whereas another with the same problem will require investigation and possibly hospital referral. Some are pleased to know that a problem can be diagnosed, whereas others prefer to hear that this or that symptom is no more than a part of normal life.

The second requirement of a decision-making model is that it recognises that no two patients are the same.

Doctors

Doctors are as much individuals as are their patients. Their professional beliefs about the goodness of different approaches to health care are also influenced by their own personal experience as patients or parents or relatives and as third-party observers of the interaction between medicine and society. They have had different experiences as students and their postgraduate training is (fortunately) still not totally uniform. Their personalities also differ. Some are extrovert, others introvert. Some are more secure and can tolerate uncertainty relatively comfortably while others are by nature more anxious. Experience (personal as well as professional) and education do have the potential to change the way doctors behave. But substantial differences between doctors in how they perceive and practise their work are (again fortunately) likely to resist attempts to standardise clinical practice.

Patients, of course, recognise differences between doctors and use these to their own purposes. Accordingly, some of the polarisations between doctors (interested in children or the elderly; good or not good with psychological problems) are artificially exaggerated. All these realities make the discipline hard to research and teach and any generally usable framework or model of the consultation has to be more - rather than less - permissive or flexible.

Continuity

The last background issue to be considered is that of continuity of care - within one doctor, between colleagues in a practice and between general practice and hospital. Continuity must be thought of across long periods of time as well as within relatively discrete episodes of illness. Health and illness must also be seen as affecting families and not only the individual who is officially 'ill'.

There is legitimate criticism of the episodic nature of much contemporary general practice care (and indeed of much hospital care as well). However, doctors will always go on holiday, some off-duty is a necessity, a patient's lifetime is several times longer than a doctor's working span and sharing care within a team and with hospital colleagues is often in the patient's better interests. Without in any way suggesting that poor continuity of care is other than a serious problem, I believe that because discontinuity of care is a necessary reality, the model we describe must allow for it.

In Summary

The ideal model must cater for 'illness' factors (reflecting modern beliefs but aware that 'truth' is an inconstant concept) for 'patient' factors (which vary with time, within and between families and within and between cultures) and 'doctor' factors (which again vary over time and are influenced by experience, education and the personality of the doctor). The model must recognise that general practice is a discipline drawing its base of knowledge and range of skills and values from both biomedical and behavioural sciences. Finally, the model must recognise that each consultation is a single frame in the long-running film of a patient's lifetime, on the one hand unique but on the other hand set in a context much larger in scale than most doctors can easily comprehend.

THE MODEL

The model is better presented as a series of ideas than as a single diagram. The individual steps are self-contained and each is already (or almost) part of the established folklore of general practice work. The utility of the model lies in the way the parts are added together and the subsequent potential for the user to build in whatever further dimensions are necessary at a particular time.

The Place of General Practice in the Spectrum of Health Care

The Horder and Horder (1956) model of the way general practice services are provided and used is widely known and has proved useful over three decades. It is shown as Figure 1a. General practice services cater for some one quarter of the perceived illnesses of the

British community and somewhere between five and ten percent of these are referred for a specialist opinion or for hospital care. Figure 1a is, of course, limited by rigidity and weakened by being based on the implicit assumption that 'patients' arrive in the diagram at a uniform stage in the development of disease. These limitations matter less when the model is used to discuss the differences between general practice and hospital medicine and how the boundary between them should be drawn. They matter more when thinking more broadly (as we are now required to think) about the interface between biomedical and social science. The WHO definition of health as 'the state of complete mental, physical and social well-being and not merely the absence of illness' is useful but limited in making no comment on either inter- or intra-cultural differences in the levels at which well-being is perceived to be present or absent. If illness is re-defined as being present when 'departures from the state of complete mental, physical and social well-being become a problem for the patient', then the study of how patients decide to enter the sphere of Figure 1a becomes a science in itself. The importance of considering the 'social science' determinants of the behaviour of doctors and patients requires the re-drawing of Figure 1a as Figure 1b to remind the user of the model of the substantially permissive and even arbitrary context in which the work of general practitioners has to be viewed.

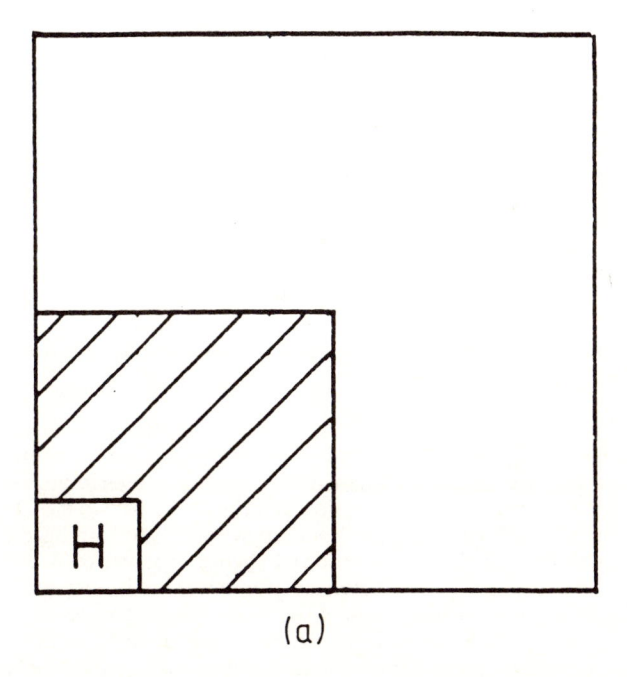

(a)

Figure 1(a) General practice services (shaded) lying between self-care and hospital services (H).

(b)

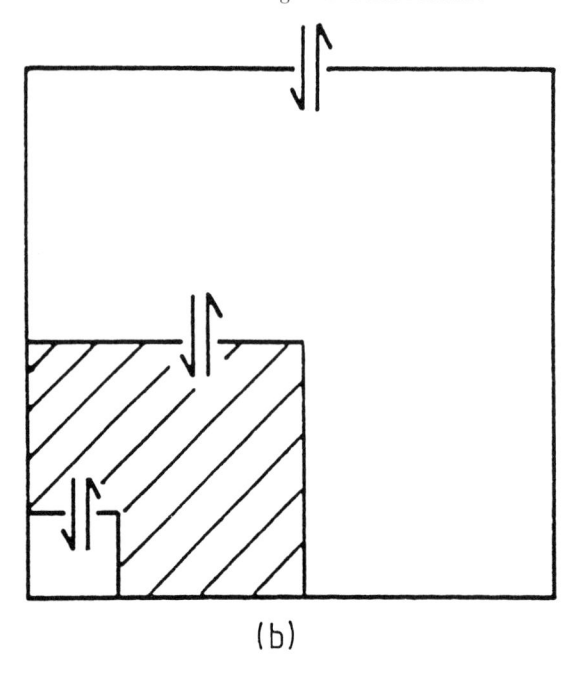

Figure 1(b) Figure 1(a), implying fluidity of patient movement within caring services.

The Perspective of the Individual Consultation

An average lifetime now covers about seventy years and the average patient has three consultations of, at best, ten minutes each with his family doctor each year. Thirty-five hours a lifetime, perhaps doubled or quadrupled to cover the family as well as the patient, implies a much smaller area of overlap between the lives of doctors and their patients than some teachings might suggest. The difficulty of simultaneously understanding consultations as single and in the context of a lifetime becomes apparent.

Figure 2a outlines a hypothetical graph of the physical ill-health of a patient over a long period of time. Figure 2b outlines a similar graph in respect of psychosocial ill-health. Figure 2c superimposes the two previous figures. A consultation taking place at time A could be viewed in several different and defendable ways. Depending on the nature of both the physical and psychosocial symptoms, it could be argued that the physical illness had caused psychosocial illness or the reverse, or that the increases in each, though associated, were not related. In deciding management, it could be in order to forecast improvement in either or both components of the illness and take no action; it would equally be reasonable to attempt to modify the natural history of either part of the illness by drug or other therapy if the doctor judged that the potential benefits of treatment outweighed the

The Consultation: A Multi-Purpose Framework 7

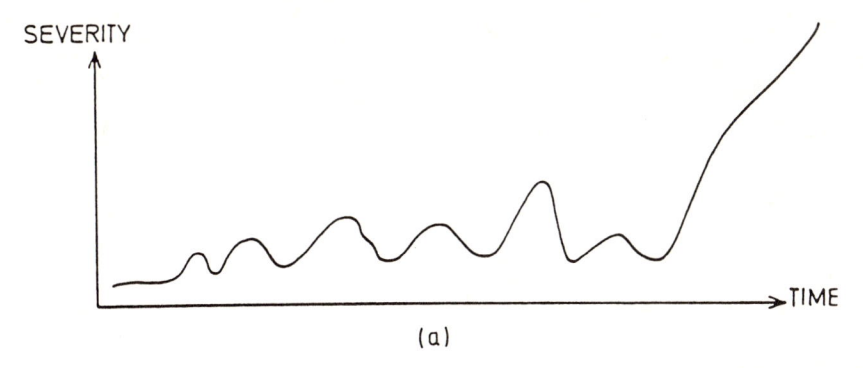

Figure 2(a) Hypothetical graph of severity of physical ill-health over a period of time.

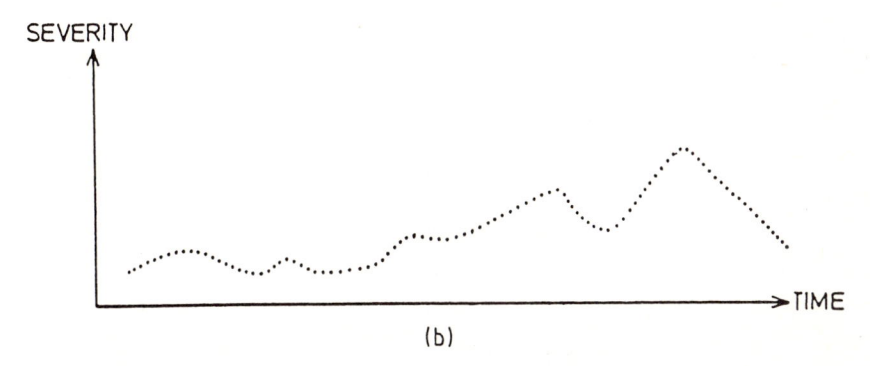

Figure 2(b) Hypothetical graph of level of psychosocial ill-health over the same time as figure 2(a).

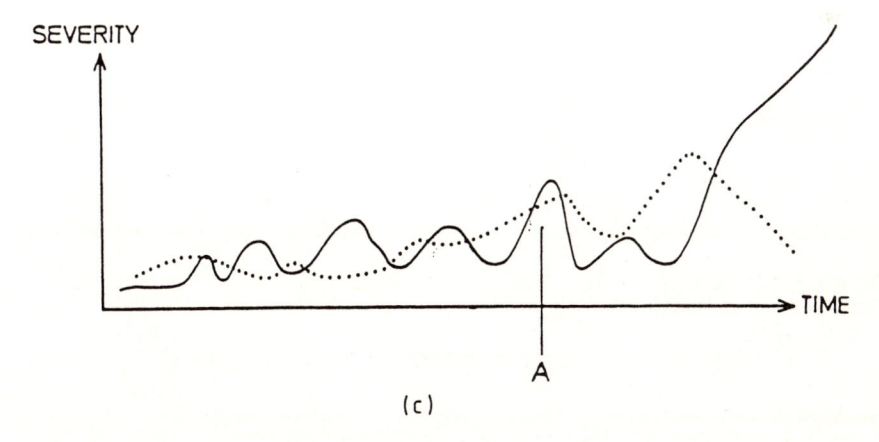

Figure 2(c) Hypothetical relationship between physical and psychosocial ill-health in one patient over a period of time.

risks (both of treatment and of 'inactive' observation). The information available to the doctor making the decision is much too substantial and complicated to be listed; the information he actually uses is more accessible to discussion and categorisation. At the next consultation, whether days or years later, he has available the additional knowledge of what has happened since the last occasion and a 'better' decision may be possible. Differences in experience, in judgement and in knowledge of the patient/family will result in different decisions being taken. Whether these decisions can be sub-divided into right and wrong is another matter. Occasionally it will be possible, usually not.

If the first part of the model is about seeing ill-health in the context of medical services, this second part is about seeing it in the context of the patient's life.

Within the Consultation

The conduct of an individual consultation is an interaction of three components. Two are people, namely the doctor and the patient; the third is the problem under discussion, or 'the illness'. The three components can be thought of as inter-relating as shown in Figure 3a. Often the context has to be broadened to include the wider implications of family practice as against general practice as in Figure 3b. Poor medicine - let alone poor general practice - centres on the diagnosis and management of the illness in isolation; the better the medicine, the greater the involvement of patient factors and the greater the use of doctor factors to develop the fullest possible inter-relationships between all the elements shown in Figures 3a and 3b.

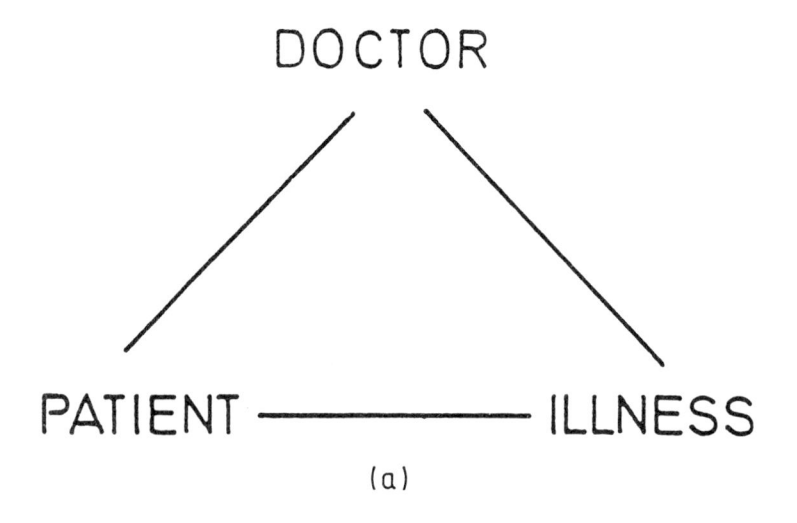

```
            DOCTOR
            /    \
           /      \
          /        \
         /          \
   PATIENT ———————— ILLNESS
              (a)
```

Figure 3(a) Principal component elements involved in any medical consultation.

```
              DOCTOR
              /    \
             /      \
            /        \
           /  FAMILY   \
          /            \
         /              \
    PATIENT ──────────── ILLNESS
              (b)
```

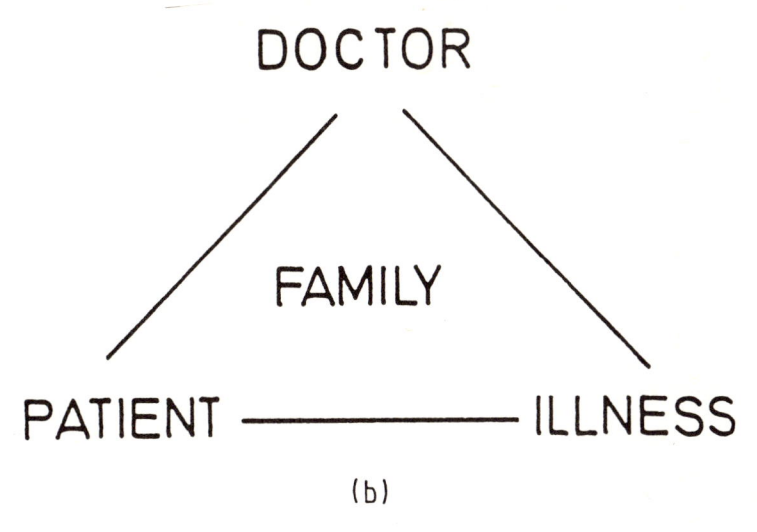

Figure 3(b) Component elements in Figure 3(a), placed in general practice context.

Consultations differ enormously in their complexity and significance, some being remarkably straightforward, others so involved that no clear beginning or end point can be determined. Any model that would set out to pre-determine the outcome - or even the structure - of a consultation in directive terms must be a denial of the uniqueness of patients and doctors, the reality of clinical judgement, and the belief that good medical care is a true art. Equally, a model that does not lay foundations for deepening the perceptiveness and broadening the scope of a consultation will be educationally, clinically and analytically impotent. To the simple framework I have proposed, additions can be made as needed and appropriate. 'Illness' can be sub-divided into physical, psychological and social; 'patient' includes age and sex differences that are relatively objective but also, for example, social class, cultural and personality differences that may outweigh in importance some of the distinctions between whether a respiratory illness is called influenza or otitis media. 'Doctor' variables are equally important and will at least include knowledge and skill as well as once again personal, personality and cultural attributes. The sub-definitions of 'family' are again many and the relevant list can be visualised as the occasion requires.

ITS DEFENCE AND ITS USES

It is, of course, only possible to 'prove' that a framework does not explain a process adequately. The more complex the framework, the more likely it is that it will fail to be universally acceptable. For those who believe in uniformity and standardisation, the outlines I have presented will seem mischievously permissive, because they do in truth appear to allow the defence of almost any decision the doctor chooses to take at a consultation.

Clinical freedom is a responsibility and not a right. The intellectual freedom to think expansively must be married with the practical discipline of critical evaluation of the consequences of decisions taken. The need to defend a decision rests particularly heavily on the doctor who chooses policies which attract only minority support from his colleagues. At the same time, the substantial absence of clear indices of benefit for one approach to care against another means that those who choose to differentiate right from wrong risk accusations of arrogance.

This is true even when wholly clinical outcomes are compared; how does one compare four days pain with untreated tonsillitis but no risk of penicillin allergy against three days of pain with (penicillin) treated tonsillitis and a 1:1000 risk of penicillin allergy? The additional issue of risk of development of rheumatic fever or acute nephritis is quantifiable only in approximate terms (Taylor and Howie, 1983) and clearly has varied with time, with social conditions and in different countries.

The doctor who prescibes antibiotics for sore throats probably creates patient expectations when lead to higher consultation rates (Howie and Hutchison, 1978). Is doctor-dependence an illness and what are its wider implication on health perception and behaviour? The widely different way patients are known to perceive and present illness owes at least something to how doctors have conditioned them - and conditioning extends across families and across generations.

Antibiotic prescribing (as measured in simulated conditions and observed in reality) for standard clinical respiratory presentations is apparently influenced by social and psychological features of the patient consulting (Howie, 1976). Where the risks of unfavourable reaction to therapy are low, how can they be compared to the patient-values of satisfied expectations or allayed anxieties. How does the conflict created by dispute between doctor and patient over an issue such as antibiotic prescribing carry over to affect future health care of the immediate patient presenting, or of the next patient due to be seen by the now-stressed doctor?

Finally, does the doctor who treats the mother's anxiety as more important than the child's catarrhal illness attract praise or criticism - and how much of either? (Howie and Bigg, 1980)

It is relatively easy to argue that a high overall antibiotic prescribing rate for respiratory illness is now harder to justify than is a low prescribing rate. This can be done in clinical terms and in behavioural terms. However, correctness for the individual patient must still be argued uniquely and the point of balance will vary from doctor to doctor as matters such as confidence and experience interact with factual knowledge and consulting skill.

I believe my model is compatible with all the realities, beliefs and caveats these last paragraphs have stated and raised. Once again, as long as the concept of clinical freedom being a responsibility is accepted, the framework seems safe and constructive.

Its Uses

Doctors work as clinicians, teachers, researchers and planners. The roles overlap substantially, although at any one time one or more will dominate. All clinicians have had consultations leading to a clearly unsatisfactory outsome. I believe the clinician learns best from analysing his own successes and failures but needs to be able to do so against a structure. The one I have described is the one I use. It helps during a consultation as well as in retrospect. Bad consultations result from having insufficient clinical knowledge, from failing to relate to patients or from failing to understand the patient's behaviour (Figure 1), his perception of his illness (Figure 3) or its context (Figure 2).

Teachers and researchers only embody different aspects of the roles of clinicians. In each role there is a need to stand back and analyse. The more logical and perceptive the analyses, the more useful they are. Analysis should lead to the ability to synthesise. Education and planning rely on synthesis taking place using sound principles on sound foundations. Again I have found that my work in all three of these spheres has been assisted by the structured approach to analysis and synthesis I have described. In the end, I believe right and wrong will come to be seen more as judgements of the way doctors think about and discuss their work than in terms of what they are actually seen to do.

CONCLUSION

Early in my time in general practice, I saw the absence of definition of the discipline and how to work in it as a fault requiring change. Being involved in the process of definition encouraged me to form an early belief that conformity was a desirable aim. The challenge facing 'academicness' in general practice is to pursue the first challenge without falling into the trap of the second.

Feinstein (1972) wrote 'until the methods of science are made satisfactory for all the important distinctions of human phenomena, our best approach to many problems in therapy will be to rely on the judgements of thoughtful people who are familiar with the total realities of human ailments'. All thoughtfully involved in general practice - whether 'academic' or not - need some framework against which to test and develop themselves and their discipline, and I have presented and defended the one I use.

REFERENCES

Aitchison, J., Brown, J.J., Ferris, J.B., Fraser, R., Kay, A.W., Lever, A.F., Neville, A.M., Symington, T., Robertson, J.I.S., (1971), 'Quadric Analysis in the Pre-Operative Distinction between Patients with and without Adrenocortical Tumors in Hypertension with Aldosterone Excess and Low Plasma Renin,' American Heart Journal, 82, 660-671.

de Dombal, F.T., Horrocks, J.C., Staniland, J.R., Gill, R.W., (1971a), 'Simulation of Clinical Diagnosis - A Comparative Study,' British Medical Journal, ii, 575-577.

de Dombal, F.T., Horrocks, J.C., Staniland, J.R., Guillon, P.J., (1971b), 'Production of Artificial 'Case-Histories' by Using a Small Computer,' British Medical Journal, ii, 578-581.

Feinstein, A.R. (1967), 'Clinical Judgement,' Williams and Wilkins, Baltimore.

Feinstein, A.R. (1972), 'The Need for Humanised Science in Evaluating Medication,' Lancet, ii, 421-423.

Howie, J.G.R. (1976), 'Clinical Judgment and Antibiotic Use in General Practice,' British Medical Journal, ii, 1061-1064.

Howie, J.G.R., Bigg, A.R. (1980), 'Family Trends in Psychotropic and Antibiotic Prescribing in General Practice,' British Medical Journal, 280, 836-838.

Howie, J.G.R., Hutchison, K.R. (1978), 'Antibiotics and Respiratory Illness in General Practice: Prescribing Policy and Workload,' British Medical Journal, ii, 1342.

Taylor, J.L., Howie, J.G.R. (1983), 'Antibiotics, Sore Throats and Acute Nephritis,' Journal of the Royal College of General Practitioners, 33, 783-786.,

Taylor, T.R., Aitchison, J., McGirr, E.M. (1971), 'Doctors as Decision-Makers: A Computer-Assisted Study of Diagnosis as a Cognitive Skill,' British Medical Journal, iii, 35-40.

2
The Consultation Process

Frank Martin Hull

When the Irishman was asked the way to Dublin, he replied, "Sure, I wouldn't start from here". I have come to suspect that, in many ways, we are starting our decision-making in general practice from the wrong place.

When doctors of my generation entered general practice, often with four or five years of post-graduate experience, we were horrified at our inadequacy. We had been educated in hospital methods of data gathering and decision-making based on a partially ordered and highly selected group of patients, most of whom had serious physical illness. The shock of finding oneself confronted by huge numbers of totally disorganised, often quite insignificant problems that were as often psychological or social as they were physical was daunting in the extreme. New entrants to general practice responded in a number of ways: some found the whole business trivial and irritating - not at all what they had studied so hard to do. Others responded with despair and depression and these two groups tended to increase the view, widely held before about 1965, that general practice was for the drop-outs. However, many doctors responded by devising a survival method - a way in which they could cope with the problem of rapid decision-making. In doing this, they had to abandon many of the principles laid down in the Mosaic tablets of the medical schools. In doing so, they felt guilt: survival demanded pragmatism, and pragmatism produced a sense of unworthiness.

Crombie (1963) published a paper on decision-making in general practice. My feelings on reading this were interesting - how dare a doctor make such statements about decision-making which were not only atypical, but quite wrong. The only sensible way to demonstrate how wrong Crombie was was to repeat his experiment. Of course, you know what happened - after collecting data as he had done, I found that my results (Hull, 1969 a & b) confirmed his findings. I learned a lot about decision-making while doing that work and I learned more about myself and about the fundamental principle defined by Mark Twain, "It ain't what I don't know that makes me a fool as what I do know that ain't so."

Despite this early realisation that the pragmatic doctor's response to the challenge of decision-making in general practice was much the same wherever he was working, the guilt, born of inappropriate didactic teaching of the medical schools, remained. Probably to this day the conviction of the rightness of medical school teaching (which varies from doctor to doctor) accounts for the fact that there may be enormous variation between doctors' methods of data collection and decision-making.

The basic unassailable facts were these: there were a large number of decisions to make in a very short time. I found myself thinking of the problem posed by a single hour in which ten men with identical coughs had to be seen in an attempt to distinguish the one whose carcinoma would shortly become inoperable from the other nine whose equally trivial cough was caused by self-limiting simple infection. This depended on answering the question, what does this symptom mean in this patient at this time? Since the symptom was the same, more effort had to go into examining qualities in the patient and why he had chosen to present at that particular surgery (Hull, 1971). This led to enquiring into the attitudes held by different types of patients using such grouping as age, sex, marital state, social class, how well the patient is known and a whole host of other data absorbed from one's own knowledge or that of practice staff or even from community gossip. In such a way, one was able to develop that useful warning light, which all of us recognise, that suddenly lights up to announce that there is something unusual.

Perhaps an anecdote will illustrate what I mean. One summer a farmer patient of mine started selling off his prize Friesian herd and I noticed that he started putting his best grazing land under the plough. While I was speculating on what he was up to, I was called to see his herdsman, an uncomplaining Italian, who had 'flu, and so instantly I diagnosed my first case of Brucellosis, because the various observed facts suddenly formed a pattern.

That diagnosis filled me with considerable pride at the time, but perhaps, looking back after twenty years, one might say that we really ought not to let preventable disease like that occur and that, if a general practitioner is really doing his stuff, he should be just as aware of zoonotic hazard as of occupational disease or other preventable conditions such as stroke, many infectious diseases and some cancers. As we enter the last sixteen years of the century, we must remember that challenge posed by the W.H.O., 'Health for all by the year 2000', which requires a new attitude to symptoms and, even more important, a new attitude to patients, especially those individuals or groups who for many reasons do not report symptoms to the doctor.

Since I diagnosed that case of Brucellosis, general practice has advanced a great deal - we have moved out of the 'cottage industry' image into the modern health centre. We have taken on much greater clinical responsibility and have actually moved closer to the model constructed by our medical schools. In doing so, we have become more efficient, but at the considerable cost of becoming more officious. We have only to look at the work of Cartwright (Cartwright 1967; Cartwright & Anderson, 1981) to see that, despite many changes in general practice, the image we show to our patients is no better and often actually worse. When, ten years ago, I moved from an adapted Victorian house to a large purpose-built medical centre, a patient commented, "Very nice doctor, but will you be the same?"

In the past, we asked, "What does this symptom mean in this patient at this time?" That is no longer enough, for that question implied that the symptom had to be presented to us. Such presentation depended on there being a symptom in the first place, on it worrying or bothering the patient and on a whole series of attitudes within the patient, which influenced his decision to consult the doctor in order to have his symptom evaluated. Such a convention inevitably led to care consisting of crisis intervention, which will certainly not help us towards meeting the W.H.O. challenge.

Before, we used to look at problems which it was "proper" to offer doctors, but now we must start a great deal earlier with conditions which may not even have yet started producing symptoms. That is what I mean by questioning if we are starting from the right place.

In 1954, John and Elizabeth Horder produced their squares of disease (Horder & Horder, 1954), which I have modified slightly (Figure 1). The large square represents all the symptoms which exist in a

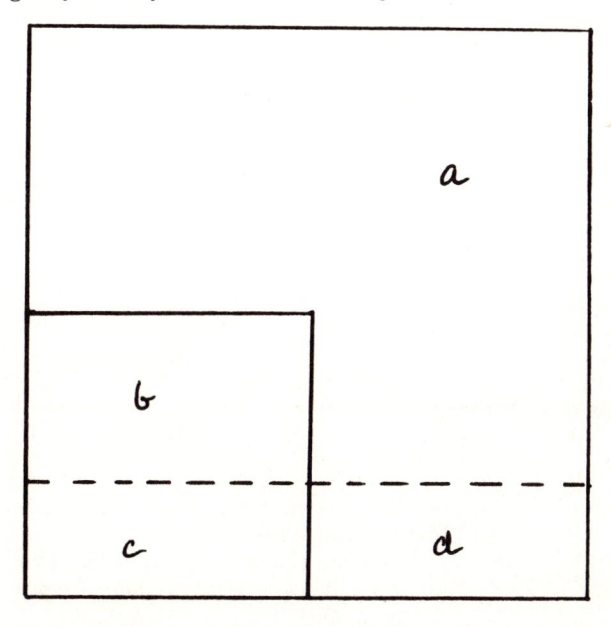

Figure 1 Square of Disease (after Horder and Horder, 1954)

given community and the smaller square, the twenty-five percent who consult their doctor. To this I have added a dotted line, quite arbitrarily placed, below which are those patients whose symptoms are significant - for example, a lump in the breast or a discharging ear - which have a high predictive value of life-threatening or crippling disease. Of course, the diagram represents the totality of symptoms - one could draw a similar diagram for, say, cough, vaginal discharge, gastrointestinal symptoms and so on.

The diagram has four areas:

(a) Those with insignificant symptoms who do not consult.

(b) Those with insignificant symptoms who do consult.

(c) Those with significant symptoms who do consult.

(d) Those with significant symptoms who do not consult.

In the past, our diagnostic effort has been largely focussed on boxes (b) and (c) with most stress on (c). Sometimes our irritation at the contact of box (b) may also have been apparent to our patients. The pathway to diagnosis used to start in the smaller square of the Horder diagram, now we have to meet the challenge of starting in box (d).

What do we know of the people who do not report their symptoms? Actually we know quite a lot. These are the people who are found dead or who report their illness just in time to get their death certificate. We get another clue to them in the patients who stop at the door at the end of the consultation and say, "By the way, does it matter if you vomit blood?", "...have a lump?" or "...can't swallow?" These are the patients who narrowly missed being in box (d) - but for every, "By the way..." symptom mentioned at the last minute, how many patients go through the door without speaking their fears? We will return to this question.

We know a good deal about certain qualities of patients who are likely to be in box (d) with certain symptoms and yet in other boxes with other symptoms. For example, we know that women of low social class, who have an increased risk of cervical cancer, are least likely to present with gynaecological symptoms. In unpublished data from a survey carried out into consultation patterns in general practice in 1970, relationships between social classes and reporting of symptoms was seen. Here the proportion of all symptoms caused by gynaecological symptoms for each social class (after exclusion of armed services) shows a gradient (Figure 2). A similar gradient is shown for eye symptoms (Figure 3) and a different one for skeletal pain (Figure 4). These may represent differences in morbidity or, as I suspect, of attitudes held by patients of different social class towards certain symptoms.

GYNECOLOGICAL SYMPTOMS

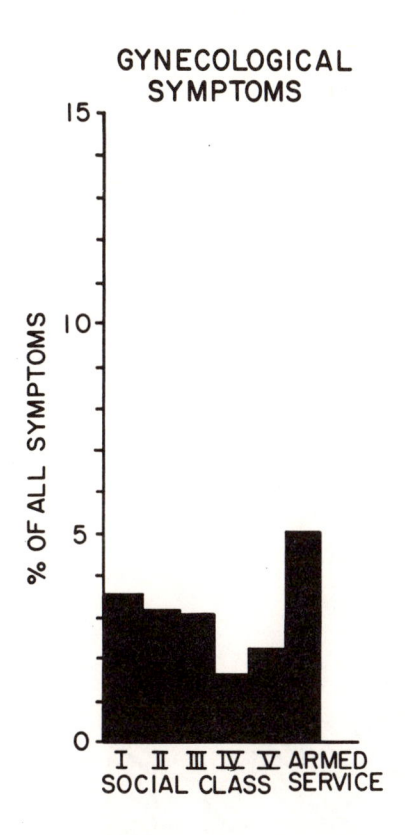

Figure 2 Gynaecological symptoms by social class. Each column expressed as a percentage of all symptoms presented in each social class. (From an analysis of 5904 new presenting symptoms in general practice)

There is another phenomenon which we have all noticed and that is that patients who see us about one, perhaps fairly insignificant symptom, may fail to mention the serious symptom that coexists. In other words, they are at the same time in both boxes (b) and (d) but with regard to different symptoms. During 1982, I gave a questionnaire (Hull & Hull, 1984) to some 1100 patients leaving their doctor's consulting room. In this questionnaire, I asked whether the patient had been satisfied that he or she had been able to communicate his/her problem to the doctor and the patient was given a five point scale marked: Not at all, A little bit, About half, Fairly well, Very well indeed. You will see (Figure 5) that many patients felt they had not told the doctor why they had come, and that when we look at the group of 355 women between the ages of fifteen an forty-five, more than half expressed reservations about whether they had really told the doctor why they had come.

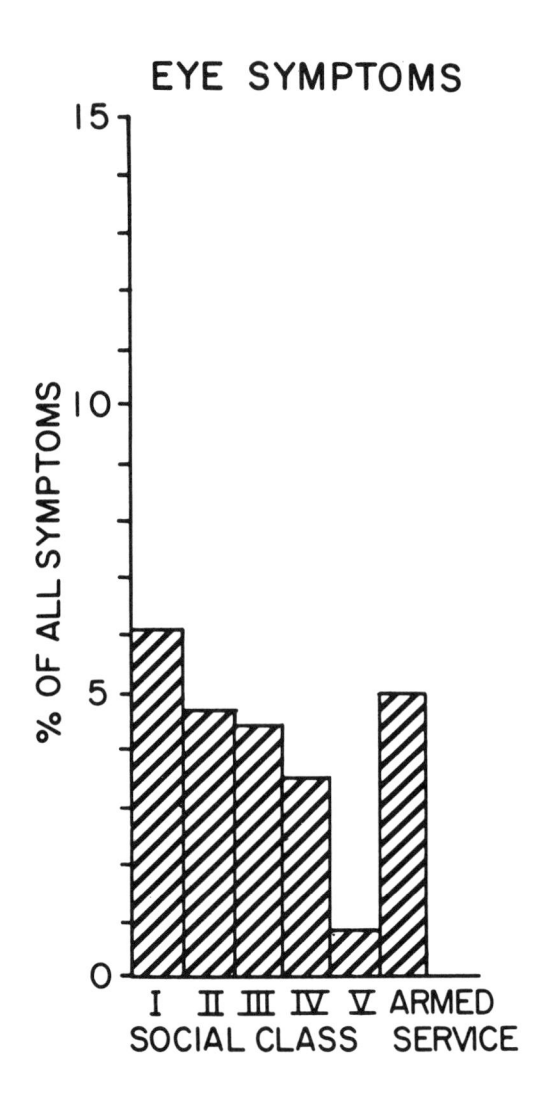

Figure 3 As Figure 2, but for eye symptoms

SKELETAL PAIN SYMPTOMS

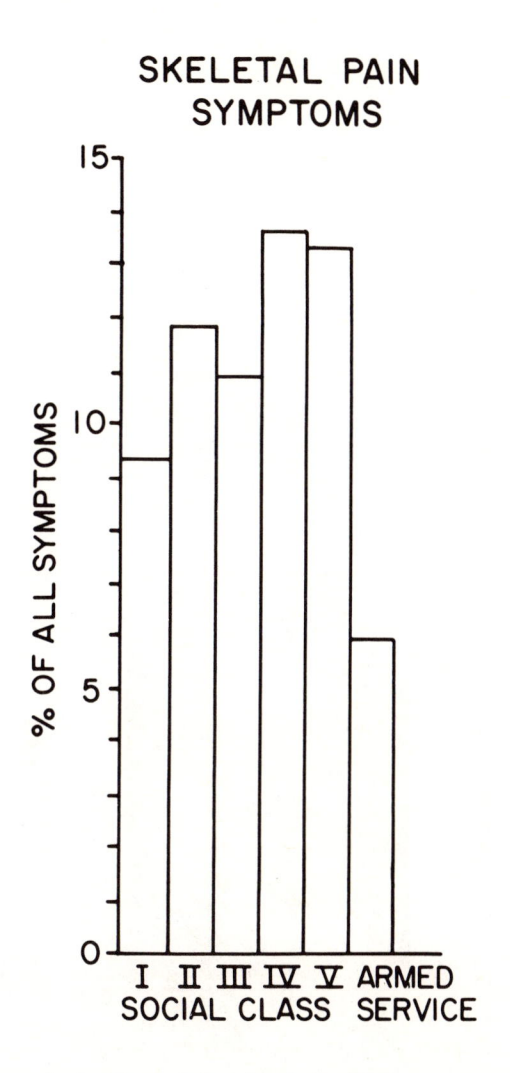

Figure 4 As Figure 2, but for skeletal pain symptoms

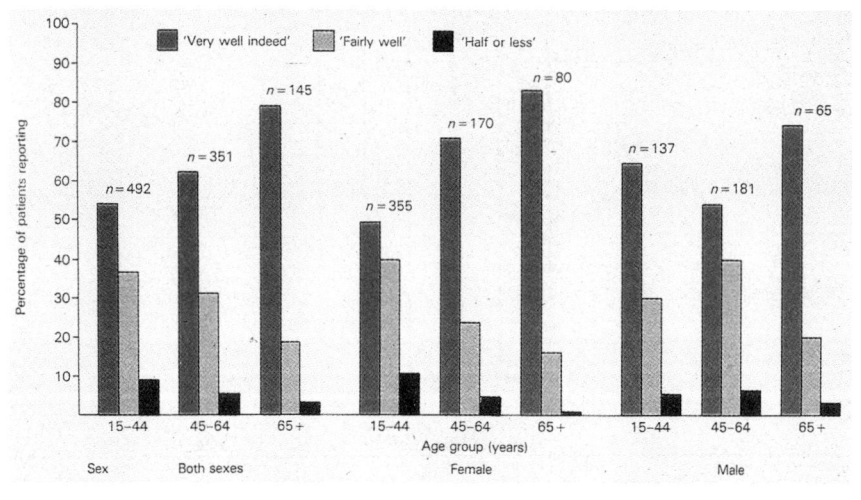

Figure 5 Patients' estimate of ease of communication with doctor in relation to age and sex

So perhaps the major improvement we can make in decision-making is easing the constraint of time and there are many ways in which we can do this, such as reduction in list size or more delegation. The coming of the computer may be of help in providing better information recall and a move to better organisation certainly helps to ease the burden of time, but both computers and better organisation are not without problems.

In the field of attitudes in the patient which influence whether or not a given symptom is presented to the doctor for evaluation, the problem of organisation is important. As we have moved out of the cottage industry into 1980s general practice, we have undoubtedly become more efficient, but have also become more officious, and this has turned off a number of patients. But the most important influencing factor in whether or not a symptom is presented, is the image of the doctor. Alas, this is all too well described in Cartwright and Anderson (1981). He is often too busy, too aloof, too cultured, too educated, too rich to be approachable by the section of the community who get the least good care. This is why, in Birmingham, we are trying an experiment (Ferriman, 1983) in an inner city practice of employing a Nurse Practitioner (Stilwell, 1982) on North American lines, to see if we can encourage patients to report symptoms early where the socio-cultural gap between them and the doctor has an inhibiting effect. In addition to coping with this effect, we need to direct much more resource into the education of under-consulting groups into how to use the available expensive medical facilities.

Lastly, what can we do about doctors? Much that my generation complained about has been and is being addressed. At least we now have general practitioners teaching in our medical schools and we are moving towards the goal of adequate undergraduate preparation for general practice. We now have vocational training so that at last the new principals in practice will not be as green as we were when we started. So far so good, but in the last few minutes of this paper I want to share with you some doubts which arise from another study at Birmingham.

Like most schools, we have a clinical introductory course in which the Birmingham General Practice Teaching Research Unit plays a large part. We teach behavioural medicine: how patients and doctors relate to each other, how patients see their symptoms, particularly with regard to their fears of disease and of what the doctors may do to them. We spend time on terminal care, on telling patients about poor prognosis and on dying and bereavement. We have assessed this for some years with a modified essay question, but you cannot, in a written paper, say, "At this point, the doctor gave the patient 'a meaningful look' - write an essay on 'a meaningful look'", and yet that is what we wanted to do after teaching about non-verbal communication.

Perhaps you begin to see why I share the Irishman's worry that we may not be starting from the right place in considering the patients' presenting symptom! And I believe that this is essential to our future thinking about decision-making in general practice.

Now, what can we do about it? It seems to me that the problem, as always, centres on time and how long we actually spend face to face with our patients - the single frame of John Howie's cine film (Howie, 1985). But there are also problems in both patient and doctor which we need to examine before we can attempt to meet the challenge of diagnosing unpresented problems.

So far as time is concerned, it is commonly believed by our patients and by ourselves that we are busy. We see our busy-ness as a virtue; patients see it in a different way: "He's too busy", "He hasn't got time to talk" and so on. But how busy are we? I asked a number of doctors to estimate how they divided the 8,760 hours of the year between sleep, various categories of work and leisure (Hull, 1983). Of course, such an estimate is soft and the results would give an impression of doctor's priorities rather than an accurate measurement, but I was surprised at how many doctors were prepared to admit that they spent little time working - some (like you, of course) work excessively. Figure 6 shows the mean of 260 doctors in fifteen countries, and that Dr. Average sleeps or plays for 60% of his time and works for 40%. That admittedly is about 60 hours which, though quite a good average compared with manual workers, is no more than other professionals. These returns came from many countries and certain aspects of work - home visiting, for example (Figure 7) - show marked differences in behaviour of doctors in the various countries. Such variations naturally reflect differences in health care systems, but also in culture which dictates attitudes and expectations. The contrast in time spent on home visiting in Belgium on one hand, and in Sweden and the United States, is most marked.

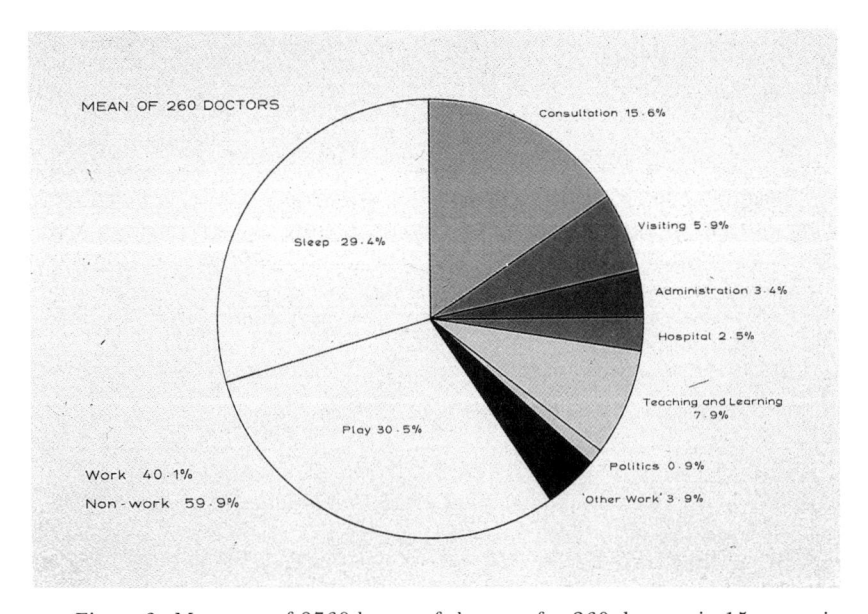

Figure 6 Mean use of 8760 hours of the year for 260 doctors in 15 countries

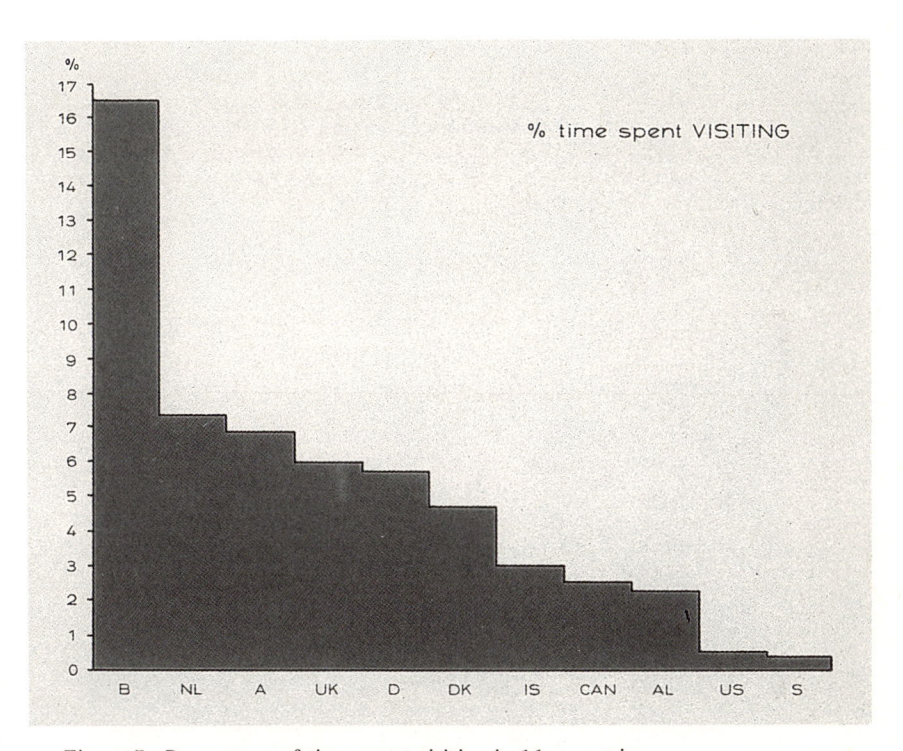

Figure 7   Percentage of time spent visiting in 11 countries

A = Austria
AL = Australia
B = Belgium
CAN = Canada
D = West Germany
DK = Denmark
IS = Israel
NL = Holland
S = Sweden
UK = United Kingdom
US = United States

But it is in consulting that the difference is most relevant to my theme (Figure 8). British doctors actually spend less time consulting than do other doctors and only about half the time that their Canadian counterparts spend seeing patients in the surgery or office. This observation, I believe, is important in its influence on decision-making in general practice.

So what of the hallowed six minutes, the mean consulting time, the single frame of Howie's cine film? Is it as so many of us protest, long enough? Patients complain of rushed, hurried doctors and this becomes more apparent in my patient satisfaction survey when appointment times are very short. Appointment times could, of course, be too long - we all know how a long interview can be emotionally draining. It may be that there is a maximum time governed by doctor efficiency, just as there may be a minimum time constrained by patient efficiency in communicating his problem.

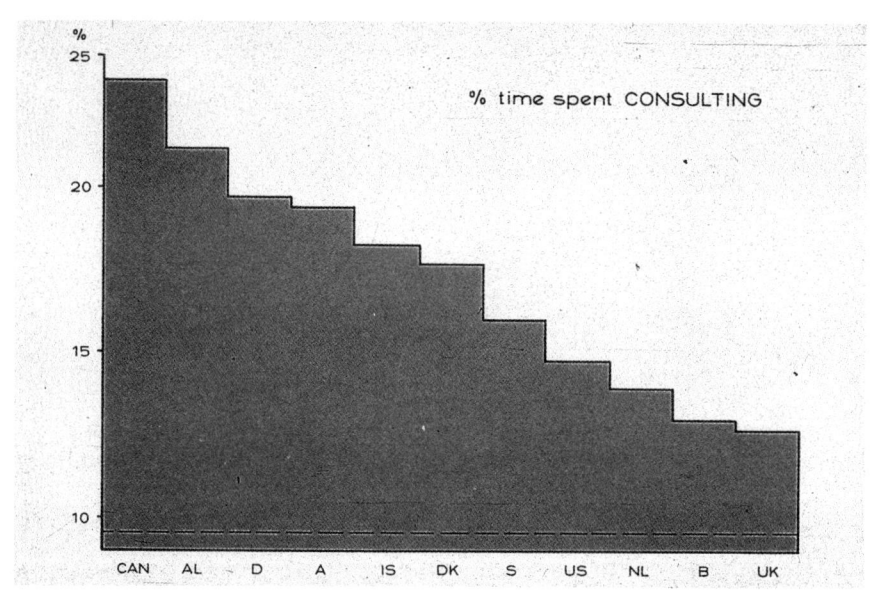

Figure 8   Percentage of time spent consulting in 11 different countries (legend as for Figure 7)

This led us to develop a video-taped examination in which students saw a case develop, in fourteen very short sequences, answering a question paper after each sequence. We now have some experience of this examination and have put it to several groups of people: students, sixth formers and doctors on completion of vocational training. The results are worrying: there is little difference in the mean mark of the three groups, and in some sections of the examination sixth formers do better than either students or vocational trainees - these parts of the examination set out to test sensitivity. This suggests that medical education, far from improving the ability of the doctor to respond to early symptoms, may actually be making matters worse. If this is so, it has enormous implications for all of us who teach medical students or who think about decision-making in general practice.

In conclusion, I would stress that the starting point for decision-making in general practice has shifted from the problem that is shown to the doctor to the problem which exists, whether or not it is shown to the doctor. This is a difficult concept, but there are ways in which we can predict such problems and as we move towards the year 2000 we must concentrate on them. We must attempt to remove barriers which prevent the early presentation of symptoms and we must educate patients to use their doctors more effectively. Lastly, we must identify and remove those aspects of medical education, both undergraduate and in vocational training, which diminish sensitivity in the next generation of doctors.

That way, I believe we may actually get to the right place to start.

REFERENCES

Cartwright, A., (1967), 'Patients and their Doctors,' Routledge & Kegan Paul, London.

Cartwright, A., and Anderson, R., (1981), 'General Practice Revisited; Tavistock Publications, London.

Crombie, D. L., (1963), 'Diagnostic Process,' Journal of the College of General Practitioners, 6, 569.

Ferriman, A., (1983), 'On the Way - Nurse who is Part GP,' Observer Newspaper, 18th May, 1983, p. 4.

Horder, J. and Horder, E., (1954), 'Illness in General Practice,' Practitioner, 173, 174.

Howie, J.G.R., (1985). This volume.

Hull, F. M., (1969a), 'Social Class Consultation Patterns in Rural General Practice,' Journal of the Royal College of General Practitioners, 18, 65.

Hull, F. M., (1969b), 'Diagnostic Pathways in Rural General Practice,' Journal of the Royal College of General Practitioners, 18, 148.

Hull, F. M. (1971), 'Diagnostic Pathways in General Practice,' Proceedings of the Royal Society of Medicine, 64, 677.

Hull, F. M. and Hull, F. S., (1984), 'Time and the General Practitioner,' Journal of the Royal College of General Practitioners, 34, 71-75.

Hull, F. M., (1983), 'The GP's Use of Time: An International Comparison,' Update, 26, 1243.

Stilwell, B., (1982), 'The Nurse Practitioner at Work,' Nursing Times, 1799.

3
Discussion of the Papers by Howie and Hull

Ann Cartwright

First I must start with a confession - I have only read the two papers for this session so my comments may overlap with some from other papers, but I have read the titles and even that is enough to alert me to the fact that I may be treading on quite a few toes. However, I think that when general practitioners invite social scientists to take part in their discussions, that is what they expect.

When I booked into a workshop on decision-making in general practice I thought I would be coming to a pragmatic discussion which would give me some insights into the day to day working of general practice. I do not use the word pragmatic in any derogatory sense. As a social scientist concerned with health and health care I go to many academic conferences where there are presentations of models and variously shaped diagrams relating to patients, their families, their illnesses and their doctors are often displayed. I thought this one would be different. I looked forward to hearing from Professor Howie and thought I might learn something more about the way doctors make their clinical judgement from further studies along the lines of his one about sore throats and the use of antibiotics.

So I was somewhat dismayed to read about his model. I must confess that I have trouble with models - to such an extent that my mind is apt to go blank (or I retreat to a fantasy world) when the term comes up. But this time, because I had to comment on the paper, I tried to stay with it. Frankly, I was unsuccessful. I cannot even make up my mind whether I am missing out on something that is altogether too subtle for me to grasp, or so simple that it seems a non-event. I hoped that in the discussion Professor Howie would explain to me how he actually uses his model. I felt I was into another fantasy world when I tried to work out what you actually did with it - besides, of course, looking at ill-health in the context of the patient's life and family and the available services when making decisions at a consultation.

I am being unfair - and over-simplifying in my turn. But to me it is a serious concern because, as I have argued before, I am worried that the academic orientation of general practitioners may be weakening their ties with patients. Previously doctors worked in comparative isolation and looked to their patients and their illnesses and social problems for professional stimulation. Now, with ancillary help, partners, University departments of general practice, trainees, postgraduate medical centres, computers and general practitioner workshops, patients have become more peripheral to the doctors' interests.

While these professional concerns and interests may have broadened the GP's perspective, improved their diagnostic and therapeutic skills and heightened their awareness of some problems, the focus of their interest has shifted. It may be now not so much on the circumstances of individual patients and of particular consultations but on how these can be fed into the computer, used to teach the trainee, to increase their reputation at the College meeting, to interest their nursing, social work and other colleagues - or be fitted into a model. An academic approach can have drawbacks for patients.

Having got that off my chest, I will turn to what I hope I am right in diagnosing as the main focus of both these papers - all the different things that need to be taken into account when making a decision in a general practice consultation. Professor Howie gives some examples of dilemmas and his model outlines the type of factors that need to be considered. Dr.Hull gives some more specific illustrations and I wholeheartedly agree with him that the people who do not consult about significant symptoms are an important consideration in relation to the conduct of consultations and the organisation of general practice.

I'd like briefly to air a bee buzzing in my bonnet about another factor which I think should be taken into account when making decisions at a consultation and that is the biased nature of the messages that a doctor is likely to be given by patients. Dr Hull has pin-pointed three biases:

    1) doctors only see patients who consult
    2) they see the frequent attenders more often
    3) and they only hear about the symptoms they select.

He also hinted at a fourth bias which is that for the most part patients express satisfactions and suppress their discontents. I know this is not always so but of course there is a bias in that you are made aware of the complaints of a vociferous minority but not about the discontents of many patients who themselves have a bias in their perceptions because they want to think well of their doctors.

The bias I want to add to this list is that patients are apt to tell you when they want something but not to mention it when they do not want it. The reason is simple : it seems gratuitous to say they don't want it before it is offered, rejecting of the doctor's help to do so afterwards. I think this often happens in relation to prescriptions - but it can also happen in relation to referrals and tests. Obviously it is important to overcome this resistance when the medicine or procedure is needed, but it is also important to avoid doing unnecessary things in the mistaken view that that is what the patient wants.

4
Patient-centred and Doctor-centred Models of Clinical Decision-making

Ian R. McWhinney

When I was given this title, my first thought was: "How many models of clinical decision-making are there?" At first sight, there appear to be many, but further reflection convinces me that many of them are variations on the same theme. My thesis will be that there are only two basic models, which I have called patient-centred and doctor-centred. In Table 1, I have listed some of the names given to these models. The names are different because they emphasize

TABLE 1 SYNONYMS OF THE PATIENT-CENTRED AND DOCTOR-CENTRED MODELS OF CLINICAL DECISION-MAKING

PATIENT-CENTRED	DOCTOR-CENTRED	
Natural	Conventional	(Crookshank 1926)
Patient-Centred	Illness-Centred	(Balint, et al 1970)
Patient-Centred	Doctor-Centred	(Byrne & Long 1976 Wright & MacAdam 1979 Stewart 1983 Levenstein 1983)
Open System	Closed System	(Stevens 1974)
Probabilistic		(Crombie 1963 Burztajn et al 1981)
High Context	Low Context	(Hall 1976)
Relational		(Carmichael & Carmichael 1977)
Holistic	Reductive	(McWhinney 1981)

different aspects of the model being described. Before I do this, let me make four general points:

(1) We should not separate clinical decision-making from the related topics of diagnosis, problem-solving, management, the doctor-patient relationship and the consultation process. Although it is possible to focus on one of these aspects only, one should do so with full understanding of the context.
Decision-making in general practice takes place within the context of the doctor-patient relationship and within the frame of the consultation. The context has an important bearing on the clinical process. The process we are discussing is one of information processing: perception, interpretation, symbolization and action. We are, therefore, concerned with everything that influences how information is perceived, interpreted, symbolized and acted on by doctor or patient.

(2) Nor is it possible to separate models of clinical decision-making from models of disease. As Crookshank (1926) pointed out, a physician's clinical method is closely related to his theory of disease. All physicians have a theory of disease, whether or not it is made explicit.

(3) All clinical methods are hypothetico-deductive, in that they involve the formulation of early hypotheses from cues presented by, or elicited from, the patient. These hypotheses are then tested by a search strategy and if necessary revised or replaced. When validated to the required level of rigour - which will vary with circumstances - the search is discontinued and certain management decisions arrived at. Brooke, Rector and Sheldon (1984) have quoted Kleinmuntz's (1968) study of neurologists as an exception to this. The subjects of this study used a series of questions to reduce the problem space in the manner of a game of 20 questions. I think we can concede that clinicains do frequently use this method and that the process is deductive. A clinician's reasoning might go something like this: "This young patient with abdominal pain is male; males do not have uteri, fallopian tubes or ovaries; therefore I need not consider ectopic pregnancy, ovarian cyst, pelvic inflammatory disease, etc.".

This process, however, can only get us so far. In most cases, we will soon come to the point where a number of alternative hypotheses must be formulated and tested. None of the aforesaid alters my view, supported by the work of Elstein et al. (1978), that clinicians work by formulating and testing hypotheses throughout the clinical process. There is nothing very unusual about this. It is the way problems are solved in all branches of science and in everyday life. Indeed, all perception is a matter of hypothesis testing (Gregory, 1977). Problems only arise if we misunderstand the nature of these hypotheses. Of course, they are not necessarily disease hypotheses. They may be hypotheses about what the problem is, or what the patient's expectations are, or what his mood is. Since the hypotheses often arise from pattern recognition, there is no conflict between pattern recognition and the hypothetico-deductive method.

(4) Each of the two models - patient-centred and doctor-centred - represents one end of a continuous spectrum, rather than a discrete and separate entity.

Ideally, a physician should be able to move easily between models during the same consultation. The findings of Byrne and Long (1976) indicate that this is the exception rather than the rule. The following statements from their book summarize their conclusions. " . . . such evidence as we have suggests that doctors have a fairly standard method of closing any consultation which in our terms has a consistent placing on the doctor/patient-centred scale". (p.105) "Our evidence leads us to conclude that the majority of general practitioners seem to evolve, largely by trial and error, a relatively static style of consulting". (p.131).
I believe that this state of affairs is due, in large part, to two causes: the dominance of the doctor-centred model in medical education, and the neglect of communication skills in the medical curriculum. As Byrne and Long (1976) remark: "The problem is that the doctor-centred style is extremely seductive." My contention will be that medicine needs a reformed clinical method and a reformed curriculum.

THE PATIENT-CENTRED MODEL

The term "patient-centred medicine" was introduced by Balint et al (1970) in contrast with "illness-centred medicine". An understanding of the patient's complaints based on patient-centred thinking was called "overall diagnosis", and an understanding based on illness-centred thinking was called "traditional diagnosis". The clinical method was described by Stevens (1974) and further elaborated by Tait (1973). Byrne and Long (1976), developed a method for categorizing a consultation as doctor or patient-centred. The concept of the patient-centred model has been further developed by Levenstein and others (1983) in work at The University of Western Ontario. The concept of a patient-centred clinical method has much in common with the psychotherapeutic concept of client-centred therapy, a term introduced by Carl Rogers (1951).

The idea of a patient-centred clinical method has actually a much longer pedigree. Crookshank (1926) pointed out that, since the origins of our clinical method in ancient Greece, there have been two meanings of diagnosis: to diagnose a disease and to diagnose a patient.

What are the features of the patient-centred model? Levenstein (Levenstein et al, 1983) has described it in the following way. In this model, the physician tries to enter the patient's world, to see the illness through the patient's eyes. He does this by behaviour which invites and facilitates openness by the patient. The central objective in every interaction is to allow the patient to express all the reasons for his attendance. The aim is to understand each patient's expectations, feelings, and fears. Every patient who seeks help has some expectations of the doctor, not necessarily made explicit. Every patient has some feelings about his problem or problems. Sometimes his feelings may be the major factor in the illness, as when a perfectly tolerable symptom is mentioned only because the patient fears cancer. Although fear is an aspect of feeling, it is such a universal component of illness that we feel justified in giving it a separate heading.

Understanding and 'tuning into' the patient's expectations, feelings and fears will be specific for each patient. Each patient's reportage of symptoms and their underlying meanings reflect his own unique world. Categorization may help the physician, but the classification of clinical phenomena, be it physical, psychological or social, comes from the doctor's world, not the patient's. It is not a substitute for the understanding of each patient as a unique individual.

The key to the patient-centred model, as its name implies, is to allow as much as possible to flow from the patient. The crucial skill is to be receptive to cues which the patient gives either verbally or non-verbally. By being receptive and listening carefully the doctor is able to take-up these cues, thereby helping the patient to express his expectations, feelings and fears.

THE DOCTOR-CENTRED MODEL

This model is so called because its main feature is the doctor's attempt to interpret the patient's illness in terms of his own explanatory framework. This means assigning the patient's illness to one of the conventional disease categories. The criterion of success is the precise classification of the illness, so that a cause may be inferred and a specific therapy prescribed. Establishing a cause includes linking the patient's symptoms and signs with organic pathology, and identifying certain causal agents such as micro-organisms.

This clinical method had its origins in the 19th century and Tait (1979) has described its evolution in the clinical records of St Bartholomew's Hospital. Structure and system first appeared in the reports of necropsies, then, about the middle of the century, in the physical examination, then, by the 1880's in the medical history. By the end of the century we had the method that still dominates medical education, a method which structures the history into Presenting Complaint, History of Present Condition, Systems Enquiry, etc.

As Tait says, this clinical method ". . . aimed to provide the student with a conceptual structure within which he could work rationally and methodically towards his goal - the formulation of a diagnosis in terms of organic pathology. For this purpose the student doctor's clinical attention was directed and made selective in character. In particular its concentration on the special points needed to achieve a diagnosis in pathological terms did result in a relative neglect of the psychological and social aspects of illness."

One might add that the pursuit of the "special points" encouraged the use of brief, short-answer, questions, and domination of the interview by the doctor.

UNIVERSALS AND PARTICULARS

Crookshank (1926) identified the differences between the two models as psychological. They represent, he maintained, two ways of thinking, two attitudes to life, two different mental sets - perhaps two personality types. One essential difference is in the attitude to particulars and universals. To the patient-centred practitioner, Crookshank's "natural diagnostician", categories are convenient concepts, explanatory models which can help us to understand a patient's illness. They are, however, man-made and subject to change as knowledge and context change. Since every illness is different in some way, the category we place it in can only fit more or less well with the illness. Moreover, an illness is such a rich and complex experience that no mere labelled category can represent more than a part of it.

The doctor-centred practitioner, Crookshank's "conventional diagnostician", has in his mind a very organized schema which he regards as having an independent reality. If put to the test, he may disclaim this, but in his clinical method he behaves as if he believes it. His method is to categorize and label the patient's disease in accordance with his schema, and to ascribe it to a specific cause.

Crookshank (1926) describes the cleavage between the two modes of thought as "between those to whom types or universals are of no greater importance than their names, or are at most but shadowy imaginings, and those to whom even the names of such types are something more than mental conveniences, algebraical symbols, or book-keeping fictions, and are representative of realities, in a Platonic if not a material sense."

Both of these methods have their strengths and weaknesses. The strength of the doctor-centred model is its explanatory and predictive power in certain types of illness. This has become more important as our therapeutic technology has become more effective. For example, the precise categorization of coronary heart disease has become more important with the advent of coronary by-pass surgery. To illustrate its potential weakness, it is illuminating to take an example from outside medicine altogether. In his book Art and Illusion, Gombrich (1960) discusses the use of formulae in the training of artists, such as the schema for drawing the human head. The problem is that the schema may so influence the artist's perception that he fails to notice the particular features of the head he is drawing. To use such a schema as the starting point can "block the path to effective portrayal unless it is accompanied by a constant willingness to correct and revise." The use of a schema should only be "a starting point which he will then clothe with flesh and blood . . ."

The parallel with medicine is striking. We use many different schemata to help us to organize and explain the data we receive from patients. These range from categories like measles, cancer of the bronchus and pernicious anaemia - relatively stable over time and in different patients - to those like tension headache, low back syndrome, unresolved grief reaction and the stages of dying. All physicians use schemata in some way. To some they are a starting point which they will then "clothe with flesh and blood"; to others they are an end in themselves, the climax of the whole process. To the doctor-centred practitioner there is a feeling of failure if he does not finish by pigeon-holing the illness into a disease category. The patient-centred practitioner knows that more than 50% of all illnesses cannot be "diagnosed" in this way. He is quite ready to reach an understanding of the illness in some other way, and this understanding can still lead to effective clinical decisions. Howie (1972) has shown how general practitioners may go from clinical observation and interpretation to treatment, without diagnosis in the conventional sense. The diagnostic label is applied post hoc, after the management decision has been made.

Another of Gombrich's images - the portrait as a useful map - is also a valuable one for us. A "diagnosis" in the patient-centred sense can be viewed as a map. The map will use certain standard schemata like contours, and symbols for roads, rivers and bridges. These symbols will be similar on all maps, but in no two maps will the relations between them be the same. The map is a "faithful construction of a relational model". Similarly with a patient-centred diagnosis, a broken leg is not just a broken leg: its significance depends on its surrounding landscape or context. To an extremely doctor-centred practitioner, however, a broken leg may be just that: a broken leg.

This brings me to two other concepts which I think are useful in differentiating between the patient- and doctor-centred models: those of mental set, and of high and low context interactions.

HIGH AND LOW CONTEXT INTERACTIONS

Cultures, subcultures, and interpersonal transactions can be classified as high, low or medium context. In high context transactions, most of the information or meaning is embedded in the external and internal contexts and very little in the universal language of the coded message. In low context transactions, the reverse is true (Hall, 1976).

A universal feature of information systems is that meaning is made up of:

1. The communication: the coded, explicit, transmitted part of the message, eg. the spoken or written communication.

2. The situation or the external context.

3. The programmed response of the recipient of the message, or the internal context. This is also referred to as the 'mental set' of the recipient.

Bernstein (1971) distinguishes between two orders of meaning: "One we could call universalistic, the other particularistic. Universalistic meanings are those in which principles and operations are made linguistically explicit, whereas particularistic orders of meaning are meanings in which principles and operation are relatively linguistically implicit. If orders of meaning are universalistic, then the meanings are less tied to a given context. ... Where orders of meaning are particularistic, ... then such meanings are less context independent and more context bound, that is, tied to a local relationship and to a local social structure. Where the meaning system is particularistic, much of the meaning is embedded in the context and may be restricted to those who share a similar contextual history. Where meanings are universalistic, they are in principle available to all because the principles and operations have been made explicit, and so public."

How does this apply to medicine? It suggests that the doctor-centred model is a low context interaction. Most of the information is transmitted in explicit coded form: the patient's description of his complaints and the physician's translation of this into his own language of symptoms and diseases. The physician is not programmed to receive inexplicit non-verbal messages and so may block out these cues. They are not part of his mental set or expectations.

The patient-centred model, it suggests, is one of a high context interaction. The meaning of the illness may be conveyed more by the context than by the coded message. This is especially likely if the doctor and patient have known each other for some time before the consultation. In this case, the doctor and patient may to some extent "share the same contextual history". Sharing the same contextual history may have great benefits, derived from the richness of communication between doctor and patient. Hall maintains that high context interactions are a way of dealing with information overload, and this may be the reason why general practice seems to be a very time efficient process. On the other hand, sharing the same context has its risks. The doctor may become so familiar with the patient, that he fails to notice changes which are apparent to an outside observer. "Missing" hypothyroidism is an example often quoted. Another risk is that the family doctor may become so much "part of the family" that he cannot take a detached view of the family's problems.

The application of these concepts to medicine are, I believe, rich in possibilities. It seems to me that our medical schools are training doctors in a low context environment where they learn a doctor-centred clinical method and acquire a mental set which blocks out much of the subtle information conveyed by patients. Internships only reinforce this training. Those who go into general practice may acquire a different mental set by a process of conversion. Some do this either intuitively or as a result of training. From what Byrne and Long (1976) have found, it appears that many do not.

VALUES

I have argued so far that the differences between the two models are psychological, and I have suggested that two important differences lie in the mental set of the physician and his attitude to universals and particulars. I now want to introduce the idea that different values underlie the two models*. In the doctor-centred model, precise categorization of the illness and attribution of cause are accorded a very high value. Precision, however, does not ensure certainty, and we are often faced with a situation in which the data are equivocal between several categories. The doctor-centred model places a high value on seeking greater precision: "leaving no stone unturned". This value is reflected in common aphorisms like: "always exclude the organic". The trouble arises when this value comes into conflict with other values, such as the safety and well-being of the patient. The risks of further investigation may be greater than the risks of implementing treatment based on the available data. Burstajn et al. (1982) give a chilling example of this value conflict in their book Medical Choices, Medical Chances. A baby was admitted to hospital because of failure to thrive and repeated infections. There was evidence of maternal deprivation and the provisional diagnosis was maternal deprivation with malnutrition and secondary immuno-deficiency. One course of action would have been to start management based on this diagnosis and treat the infant with "tender loving care", and antibiotics when required for the infections. In fact, the infant was subjected to a prolonged series of tests aimed at ruling out other causes of immuno-deficiency and identifying infecting organisms. These tests included multiple blood tests and lumbar punctures. Eventually, the infant died, and the inference is that the tests done to increase the precision of diagnosis actually contributed to its death.

---

* I am indebted to Professor Arthur Elstein and Dr John Nicholas for drawing my attention to the issues discussed in this section.

Before our present era, an excessive pursuit of precision did not carry many risks. In our own time, however, the technology of investigation has advanced so rapidly as to create many hazards, not to speak of enormous expense. Not the least of the hazards is that of finding a spurious abnormality, to which the patient's problem is attributed, with all the attendant risks of inappropriate treatment.

All this is not intended to minimize the value of appropriate precision, when it has been weighed in the balance with other values. The weakness of the doctor-centred model in its extreme form is its failure to recognize that precision is one among many values, and that greater precision does not necessarily reduce uncertainty, or lead to a more accurate definition of the problem.

In the patient-centred model, the appropriate level of precision is an important issue. Uncertainty is accepted as inevitable and the physician focuses on the evaluation of different therapeutic choices. This brings him very quickly to an inspection of the values involved. The decision about how far to go in trying to reduce uncertainty is taken against the whole context of the illness. Is there a potential weakness in the patient-centred model? The polar opposite of the excessive valuation of precision is its undervaluation. It would not be difficult to think of examples in which greater precision could have reduced uncertainty, and could have been obtained without conflicting with other values. If I seem to be biased in favour of the patient-centred model, it is not only because it is necessary for general practice, but also because I believe modern medicine to be biased in the other direction.

PROBABILITY AND DECISION-MAKING

The term "probabilistic" can be used in two senses. We can say that all perception is probabilistic. Our clinical observations of patients are probabilistic in this sense. On the other hand, we can use the term in the "Bayesian" sense. In fact there are two senses in which one can be "Bayesian"*. In the first, we are concerned with the revision of prior probabilities by using Bayes' Theorem. In the second - Bayesian Decision Theory - we are concerned with evaluating the outcome of decision alternatives as a function of probabilities and utilities.

If all perception is probabilistic then it follows that both our models are probabilistic in this sense. Even when trying to understand a patient's uniqueness, the physician is still making hypotheses based on his perceptions, and testing them by listening to what the patient says. When it comes to making clinical decisions however, I believe that the patient-centred model is Bayesian in both senses. Given a presenting symptom, the physician's ranking of

---

* I am indebted to Dr John Nicholas for this description.

hypotheses (other things being equal) will be a function of his knowledge of prior probabilities in his practice population, and of how these probabilities are altered by the symptom. We know, of course, that precise numbers are not usually attached to these probabilities. Physicians do not think in numbers. This does not alter the fact that we do think in terms of probability, or at least relative likelihood. My comment "other things being equal" expresses an important exception. Physicians will change their ranking if a disorder of low probability has a high "pay-off", eg. is life threatening and curable.

I think Howie's (1972) findings indicate that patient-centred practitioners also intuitively apply Bayesian decision analysis in the choice of alternative management strategies in conditions of uncertainty. Again, precise numbers are usually not used. It is, however, a worthwhile objective of clinical research to obtain the best possible data about prior probability, sensitivity, specificity, predictive value, risk and benefit.

The description of the clinical process in these terms has enabled us to explain why the process in general practice is inevitably different than in specialties that deal with more highly selected populations. The explanation rests on three key statements:

1) The prior probabilities of diseases and symptoms vary with the population at risk.

2) The predictive value of a test varies with the prevalence.

3) The sensitivity of a test varies with the stage of the illness.

Is the doctor-centred model Bayesian? For the same reasons, I believe that it is. If there is a difference in this respect between the two models, it is a difference in attitudes and values. In the doctor-centred model, the physician, although thinking in terms of probability, places a high value on increasing the level of probability before considering decision alternatives. In the patient-centred model, the physician is prepared to make decisions at lower levels of probability because he has considered other values.

IS GENERAL PRACTICE DIFFERENT?

I believe that general practitioners, because of the different context in which they practice, require a different mental set from that needed by physicians in other fields of medicine. Let me now summarize my reasons.

Brooke and Sheldon (1985) have pointed out that it is the nature of the problem to be solved that determines problem-solving strategy. To this I would add: it is also the perception of the problem to be solved. Perception cannot be separated from interpretation (hypothesizing). To quote Gregory (1983) ". . . the experience that one has in perception is a hypothesis". How we perceive and interpret the world is shaped by our existing mental constructs. "We see what we know." Let me give three examples of this from cognitive psychology (Bruner, Goodnow and Austin, 1956):

1) How an individual classifies data is influenced by his training. The broader the range of attributes he is exposed to during training, the greater the range of attributes he will use later in defining the category. For example, a person trained to distinguish oranges from non-oranges by exposing him only to exemplars with the colours midway between orange-yellow and red-orange will classify oranges differently from a person who has been exposed to the whole range. The parallel with clinical training is clear.

2) Individuals can <u>learn</u> to respond to cues. For example, men can be trained to <u>utilize</u> cues seldom otherwise used in "piercing" the mask of camouflage in aerial photographs.

3) The process of solving a problem is affected by the definition of the task. One aspect of the definition is the individual's expectations about what constitutes successful solution or successful progress in a problem-solving task. Again, the parallel with medicine is clear. How far one goes in trying to increase the probability of a diagnosis - or even what constitutes a "diagnosis" - will depend on one's definition of the task.

All these instances suggest that the "mental set" of the clinician is a crucial factor in what he perceives and how he interprets data. It suggests also that clinicians with such different mental sets as general practitioners and internists should show differences in the way they solve problems. Why is it, then, that some experimental evidence seems to contradict this? The answer is that differences in problem-solving due to differences in mental set will only emerge with certain types of problems. If one of us were to have a cardiac arrest, I would expect all the clinicians here to respond in the same way. In the comparison between general practitioners and internists done by Barrows et al (1982), the four test cases were patients with serious organic diseases presenting to the physician for the first time. The four diagnoses were: pericarditis, duodenal ulcer and depression, multiple sclerosis and peripheral neuritis. In this context, all the physicians could be expected to see as their chief task the attainment of a clinico-pathological diagnosis. In the similar study done by Smith and myself (1975) the same thing applies in two of the cases. In the third, however - a patient with depression and anaemia - differences between the two groups of physicians did begin to emerge.

I might add that none of us were really studying gneral practice, for the most significant feature of general practice is that, usually, the doctor already knows the patient. This difference in the external context within which problems are solved is likely, in my view, to lead to major differences in how problems are solved. Any experiment which controls the context is bound to iron out any difference that arises from the context.

Although Gale and Marsden (1985) do not use the term "mental set" I think their "memory structure" is close to it. They seem to be saying the same thing, ie. that what a clinician perceives, how he formulates a problem - the hypotheses he makes - are determined by his mental set, memory structure, world view. The clinicians in their study seem to me to be working at the "doctor-centred" end of the continuum. I could test this by asking them in any of the cases: "What did the clinician say about the patient's fears. What were his expectations in seeking help. How is the problem related to the events in his life? How is it affecting his life?"

There seems to be an assumption in their paper that the clinical method being used by these clinicians is appropriate and that it is also quite appropriate for the general practice method to be learned as an "add on". This is an assumption I wish to question. There is also a suggestion that the differences between the two methods is quantitative rather than qualitative. I do not think that one can describe differences of perception as quantitative. The difference is more like a difference in visual gestalt. Let me illustrate with a case vignette.

> A 19-year-old girl injured her knee while playing baseball and was admitted to hospital for surgery. When seen for follow-up by doctor A she showed weakness and muscle wasting in the leg and complained of a number of general symptoms (fatigue, sweating, pain in the neck). When doctor A suggested that she was not doing her exercises she became hostile and angry. Eventually she saw another doctor (doctor B), who found her with severe muscle wasting in the leg and still complaining of the same general symptoms. After excluding some physical causes of her symptoms, doctor B invited her to talk about the impact of her injury on her life. It turned out that the injury, by forcing her to cease her athletic pursuits, had, at a critical stage in her life, removed the main basis of her self concept. Given some insight into the problem, and the opportunity to discuss it with the doctor, she made a gradual recovery from her illness and returned to full activity.*

I give this case as an example because it was one in which the two doctors perceived the same problem quite differently. Doctor A saw a hostile, uncooperative and ungrateful patient with an injured knee.

---

* I owe this example to Dr Eric McCracken.

Doctor B saw a patient with an injured knee and a life crisis. I do not think that one can describe these differences as quantitative. The two doctors saw different meanings in the illness. One saw only the figure, the other the figure and the ground.

If the problem is differently perceived, then the definition of the task will be different. And if this is so, the decisional task will be differently perceived. Decision analysis has to begin after formulation of different interpretations of the problem and of different decision alternatives.* In the matrix in Figure 1, the decision alternatives (D.A.) are on the vertical axis and problem formulations (P.F.) are on the horizontal axis. In the interstices are the outcomes for each decision alternative, given each interpretation of the problem. My contention is that the range of interpretations and the range of decision alternatives will be

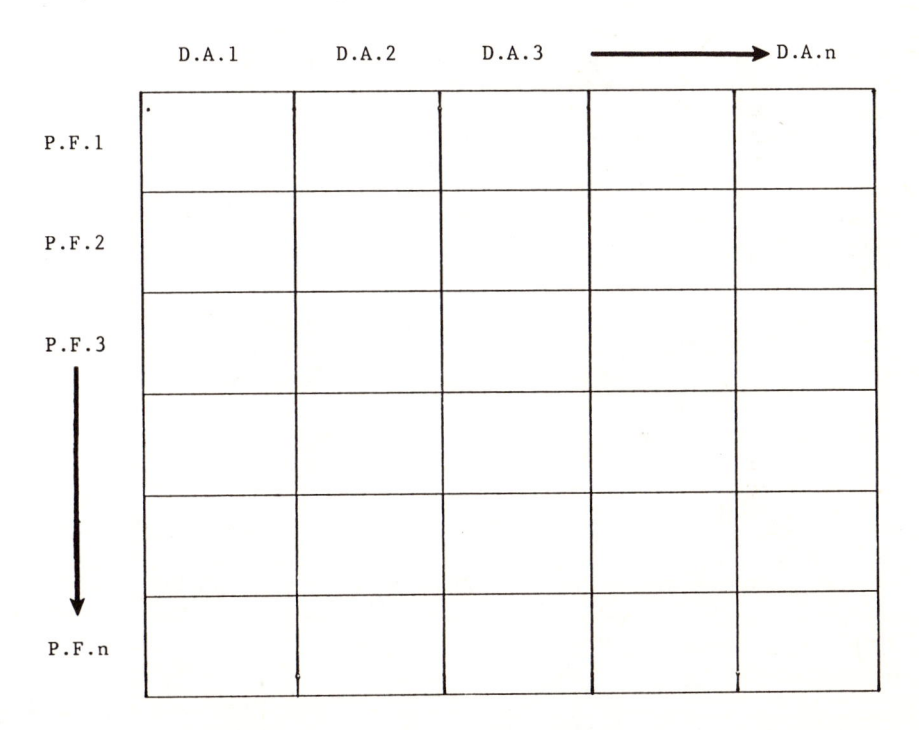

P.F. = Problem Formulation

D.A. = Decision Alternative

FIGURE 1   THE NECESSARY CONDITION FOR DECISION ANALYSIS: FORMULATION OF THE PROBLEM AND LISTING OF THE DECISION ALTERNATIVES

* I am indebted to Dr Touw-Otten for this observation.

different in the two clinical methods I have described. In the above example, doctor B was able to provide a greater variety of problem formulations and a larger choice of decision alternatives.

SUMMARY AND CONCLUSIONS

I have described two models of the clinical process, both of which rely on hypothesis testing. Bayesian probability theory and decision theory can be applied to both. Where they differ is in their objectives and in the attitudes and values that underlie them. In short, the patient-centred model focuses on diagnosing the patient, the doctor-centred model on diagnosing the disease. The two models differ in their attitude to uncertainty and to the value placed on precision, classification and causal inference.

I believe that medicine, having been dominated for many years by the doctor-centred model, is on the threshold of a major revision of its clinical method. This change is needed to adapt to a changing pattern of morbidity, to developments in technology and to changing expectations of patients. The new clinical method must assimilate behavioural science, just as the method we have inherited from the 19th century assimilated the sciences of pathology, chemistry and physiology. It must bring together the doctor- and patient-centred models, so that illnesses may be understood, not only in mechanistic terms, but also in terms of their meaning for the patient.

I believe that general practice is at the leading edge of this change. This is why the virtual exclusion of general practice from many medical schools, and the unreformed state of medical education, is such a serious matter.

Acknowledgements

I am grateful to Professor Arthur Elstein and Doctors John Nicholas, Martin Bass, Carol Buck, Moira Stewart, Eric McCracken, Wayne Weston and John Biehn for many helpful comments on early drafts of the manuscript.

REFERENCES

Balint, M., Hunt, J., Joyce, D., Marinker, M., and Woodcock, J., (1970): Treatment or Diagnosis: A Study of Repeat Prescriptions in General Practice. J. B. Lippincott Company, Toronto.

Barrows, H.S., Norman, G.R., Neufeld, V.R., and Feightner, J.W. (1982): The Clinical Reasoning of Randomly Selected Physicians in General Medical Practice. Clinical and Investigative Medicine, 5, 1, 49-55.

Bernstein, B., (1971): Class, Codes and Control. London, Routledge and Kegan Paul.

Brooke, J.B., & Sheldon, M.G., (1985): Decision = Patient with Problem + Doctor with Problem. This volume.

Brooke, J.B., Rector, A., and Sheldon, M.G., (1984): A Review of Studies of Decision-Making in General Practice. Medical Informatics, 9, 45-53.

Bruner, J.S., Goodnow, J.J., and Austin, G.A. (1956): A Study of Thinking. New York, John Wiley.

Burztajn, H., Feinbloom, R.I., Hamm, R.M., and Brodsky, A., (1981): Medical Choices, Medical Chances. New York, Delacorte Press/Seymour Lawrence.

Byrne, P.S., and Long, B.E.L., (1976): Doctors Talking to Patients. H.M. Stationery Office.

Carmichael, L., and Carmichael, J., (1982): The Relational Model in Family Practice. Marriage and Family Review 4, 123-133.

Crombie, D.C., (1963): Diagnostic Methods. The Practitioner, 191, 539.

Crookshank F.G., (1926): The Theory of Diagnosis. Lancet, ii, 939-942, 995-999.

Elstein, A.S., Shulman, L.S., and Sprafka, S.A., (1978): Medical Problem-Solving. An Analysis of Clinical Reasoning. Cambridge, Harvard University Press.

Gale, J., and Marsden, P., (1985): Diagnosis: Process not Product. This publication.

Gombrich, E.H., (1960): Art and Illusion. Princeton University Press.

Gregory, R., in Miller, J., (1983): States of Mind. British Broadcasting Corporation.

Hall, E.T., (1976): Beyond Culture. New York, Doubleday and Co.

Howie, J.G.R., (1972): Diagnosis - the Achilles Heel? Journal of the Royal College of General Practitioners, 22, 241-258.

Kleinmuntz, B., (1968): The Processing of Clinical Information by Man and Machine. In Formal Representation of Human Judgement. B. Kleinmuntz, ed. New York, John Wiley.

Levenstein, J.H., McCracken, E., Stewart, M., Brown, J., and McWhinney, I.R., (1983): A Model for the Office Visit in Family Medicine. Unpublished paper, The University of Western Ontario.

McWhinney, I.R., (1981): An Introduction to Family Medicine. New York, Oxford University Press.

Rogers, C., (1951): Client-Centred Therapy. Cambridge, Mass. Riverside Press.

Smith, D.H., and McWhinney, I.R., (1975): Comparison of the Diagnostic Methods of Family Physicians and Internists. Journal of Medical Education, 50, 264-270.

Stevens, J., (1974): Brief Encounter. Journal of the Royal College of General Practitioners, 24, 5-22.

Stewart, M.A., (1983): What is a Successful Doctor-Patient Interview - A Study of Interactions and Outcomes. Social Science and Medicine, in press.

5
A 'Model' for the General Practice Consultation

Joseph H. Levenstein

INTRODUCTION

The general practitioner (GP)-patient interaction is recognised as the cardinal feature of general practice. It is accepted that 'what happens between doctor and patient' is central to all the characteristics of the discipline. There is clarity about the problems that may emerge from the interaction, (eg. physical, psychological, social, familial, continuing and fragmentary), and the opportunities that these offer for different types of care and interaction, particularly on a continuing basis. There is also some consensus on the way the GP responds and acts on defined problems by means of the problem-solving method. Little unanimity exists, however, on the clinical method a GP uses while searching for and identifying these problems. In fact, it is well recognised that GPs vary markedly in their approach to patients.

The lack of a distinctive 'model' for general practice hampers the progress of the discipline in several ways. For example, as GPs are using different models it is understandable that morbidity studies in the discipline are often at great variance with one another. Furthermore, in the teaching of the discipline the absence of a model makes the learning, teaching and evaluation of the consultation extremely difficult and the wide variation of the trainers' models makes the exercise highly subjective. The principal objective of any interaction should be to establish the reasons for the patient's attendance. Failure to do so results in a high cost both for the patient, (failure to 'get better') and on the health care system, (repeated attendances to the doctor and unnecessary investigations). Yet it is common that this objective is not reached in a high percentage of interactions. Hull (1985) observed that more than half of 335 women between the ages of 15 and 45 years expressed reservations as to whether they had told the doctor why they had consulted. Practitioners also appear to focus on one problem only (Bentsen, 1980; Brooke and Sheldon, 1985) whereas an average of 2.7 problems were identified in videotaped interactions. Finally, each interaction takes on a further significance when we realise that the average time the GP will spend with a patient by the time he reached 70 years of age is only 35 hours (Howie, 1985).

It is argued that in general practice we should use a patient-centred model as opposed to a doctor-centred model. This means that the doctor sees each patient as a unique individual with a unique illness. He endeavours to enter and 'tune into' the patient's world and facilitate the expression of his perceptions of his illness. The doctor does not place a value judgement on the patient's illness, recognising that, whatever its nature, it is causing the latter pain and anxiety. It is also accepted that the doctor cannot be patient-centred unless he is aware of self and is prepared to make the changes in attitude and behaviour needed for such an approach.

With the above facts in mind I attempted to analyse and develop my 'model' in the doctor-patient interaction. To this effect I audio-taped about 1000 of my consultations over a period of eighteen months. Later the 'model' was further developed, taught, evaluated and researched at the University of Western Ontario on visiting Professorships in 1981 and 1982.

GENERAL PRACTICE 'MODEL'

The essence of the general practice model is to allow the patient to express all the reasons for his attendance. The aim is to understand and meet each patient's expectations, 'feelings' and fears. Every patient who seeks help has explicit and implicit expectations of the doctor. Furthermore, he has 'feelings' related to his illness, which can be as a result of several factors. Although 'fears' are 'feelings' they are such a universal component of illness that they are given a separate heading.

EXAMPLES OF DOCTOR AND PATIENT-CENTRED INTERVIEWS

Examples of patient-centred and doctor-centred interviews are presented. These simple interactions will serve to illustrate the principals of the model.

Patient-Centred Interaction

Expectation

Patient: I have this pain in my stomach

Doctor: Tell me about it ...

Patient: It's right in the middle of my stomach and it burns me ... every night

Doctor: ... every night?

Patient: Yes, just before I go to sleep

Doctor: Why do you think that is?

Feelings

Patient: I'm not quite sure but I'm having difficulty to fall asleep as well

Doctor: Mmm

Patient: It's so annoying

Doctor: What is?

Patient: All these hassles with Ted and the children, I just can't cope.
I feel hopeless and now my stomach too ...

Fears

Doctor: What about your stomach?

Patient: I was so worried I might have an ulcer

Doctor: ... and now?

Patient: Well I'm not so sure because it just comes on when I go to bed and have to face Ted. He really doesn't understand how difficult the children really are ...

Doctor-Centred Interaction

'Expectations'

Patient: I have this pain in my stomach

Doctor: We know you are having problems at home, it's your nerves

Patient: It burns. It can't be my nerves

Doctor: I'm sure it's your nerves

Patient: I can feel it in the middle of my stomach, I'm not imagining it.

'Feelings'

Doctor: No one says you're imagining it. It's caused by your nerves

Patient: If it's my nerves I must pull myself together. I didn't mean to waste your time

Doctor: Here, take these tablets

'Fears'

Patient: Can't I have an X-ray?

Doctor: You don't need an X-ray. Just take the tablets and we'll see

Patient: I suppose you know best but my stomach really burns

Doctor: You don't need an X-ray because your pain is typically 'nervous' in character

Patient: I'm sorry doctor to trouble you. Thank you.

'EXPECTATIONS'

The consultation is initiated by the patient either stating his expectation or it may be implicit such as in a doctor-initiated interaction as for a blood pressure check, for example. The patient requires his expectation to be met, regardless of whether this is his 'actual reason for attending'. If he states he has a pain in the stomach this problem should be addressed. Thus the spontaneous conscious reasons the patient presents to the doctor imply certain expectations from the doctor. The expectations are usually 'physical' in nature and relate to organs, systems or symptoms emanating from them. The doctor's response can be in the form of acknowledgment, by obtaining clarification, asking appropriate questions, performing examinations and initiating investigations, for example, with the ultimate objective of making a diagnosis and instituting treatment. Thus the doctor responds to the patient on a reality level.

Failure to meet the patient's expectations can result in a disjointed, dysfunctional interview. While in the 'doctor-centred' interaction, the physician may be quite correct in his assumptions, he has not met the patient's expectation and has imposed his perceptions on the patient with the resultant discord.

'FEELINGS'

The emotional content of the patient's illness can be reflected by the patient's 'feelings'. These may reflect the predominant part of the illness or be one of it's constituent parts. 'Feelings' are not often explicitly articulated by the patient. They are often 'under the surface' and may even be in the unconscious only surfacing during the process of the interaction. They may arise directly out of the stated expectation or may be indicative of the patient's personality, his past or way of life or his defence mechanisms for example. Often the patient requires permission to present his 'feelings'. 'Feelings' or emotions per se need not be stated directly. In the patient-centred article some are made explicit, ("I feel hopeless") or they may be implicit, (..."he doesn't understand" - indicating hopelessness and frustration). Feelings can be explored to the level the patient leads the doctor to. In the doctor-centred interview the doctor by not meeting the expectation never elicited 'feelings' related to the illness. By his approach he did manage to elicit 'feelings' of the patient's insecurity and uselessness for example, ("I didn't mean to waste your time" and "I'm sorry to trouble you"). Needless to say with a doctor-centred approach these were obviously ignored.

'FEARS'

'Fears' are almost universal to any doctor-patient interaction. To a greater or lesser extent the patient is dealing with the unknown and it is rare that the patient won't have anxieties or fantasies about his illness, its possible management and the effect it may have on his life. 'Fears', inasmuch as they are 'feelings', can have their source in the here and now, past events or be part and parcel of the patient's personality or life circumstances. In the patient-centred interview the patient's fears were expressed, ("I was so worried I might have an ulcer") but ignored in the doctor-centred interview, ("Can't I have an X-ray?").

Understanding and tuning into the patient's expectations, feelings and fears will be specific for each patient. Obviously each patient's reportage of symptoms and their underlying meaning reflect his own unique world. The key to the patient-centred model, as its name implies, is to allow as much as possible to flow from the patient. The crucial skill is to be receptive to patient cues which the patient gives verbally or non-verbally. The patient may be saying things, however trivial, or behaving in a specific way for important reasons, whether they be conscious or unconscious. By being receptive and listening carefully the doctor is able to take up patient cues, thereby helping the patient to express his expectations, feelings and fears. The doctor must also build bridges between himself and the patient to facilitate trust and communication.

'CUTTING OFF'

Failure to take up what the patient presents results in the doctor 'cutting off' the patient and thereby missing an opportunity to gain full insight into the patient's illness. It can also result in frustration for the patient, since the doctor is placing his own priorities above those of his patient. He is operating from his own world and imposing it on the patient. Interestingly enough the patient often gives the doctor several chances after being cut off. In the doctor-centred interview, the patient keeps cueing back to her stomach with all its meanings and fears but the doctor keeps cutting her off. Patients can give the most subtle cues which, if followed up, can result in some of the reasons for attendance.

Patient-centred

Doctor: Have you any other problems?

Patient: Not really

Doctor: Not really?

Patient: Well it's not much ...

Doctor: (silence)

Patient: Well it seems so silly, I'm not interested in sex any more

Doctor-centred

Doctor: Anything else wrong?

Patient: Not really

Doctor: Well good then. Just take these tablets ...

A 'Model' for the General Practice Consultation   53

DOCTORS FACILITATIVE BEHAVIOURS

The doctor in the patient-centred model must allow the interview to be dictated by the patient. To do this he must use verbal and non-verbal facilitative techniques of one or other nature. The questions must be open and non-directive allowing the patient to expand. As the objective is to follow up all the patient presents, reflective questions and silences can be extremely useful. To enter into the patient's world is a difficult art requiring the qualities of empathy, non-judgemental acceptance, congruence and honesty.

The doctor, in facilitating all aspects of the patient's illness does not run the risk of invading the patient's privacy. He does not probe or dig but merely invites the expression of the patient's feelings or opinions. If the patient does not wish to proceed, the doctor can 'get the message' and 'drop' the subject. The doctor only acts on what the patient gives him.

Doctor: You say you're not interested in sex any more?

Patient: No

Doctor: Would you like to discuss it?

Patient: Not just now

Doctor: Well fine, but please feel free to bring it up any time you like.

The patient-centred GP model does not exclude the reductionist model where the latter is appropriate, such as in the diagnosing or elimination of a clear cut organic entity or suspicious symptom. The formal medical model can be interspersed at any appropriate stage in the interaction. Also, the patient-centred interview must be seen in the context of the job definition of the general practitioner, namely to initiate preventive care and see to continuing care for all physical, psychological and social problems. In making management decisions he is called upon to a lesser or greater extent to apply his knowledge and skills. With this model where appropriate he involves the patient in the process of diagnosis and management alternatives. There are occasions when the urgency of a problem may require the doctor to impose his value system and priorities on the patient, e.g. a conflict between the patient's expectations and feelings and the physicians assessment of his needs. An example of this may be where a doctor suspects an acute myocardial infarction and the patient insists he only has heartburn and is "too busy" to go to hospital.

It is concluded that the patient's reasons for attendance should be facilitated and that these globally fall under the headings of 'expectations', 'feelings' and 'fears'. Furthermore, all that is offered, verbal and non-verbal, should be taken up and not cut off. The doctor should exhibit facilitative behaviours and endeavour to be aware of self. By following this model a dysfunctional doctor-centred interview could be avoided.

REFERENCES

Bentsen, B.G. (1980). The diagnostic process in Primary Care. In: Primary Care., Ed. Fry, J., Heineman, London.

Brooke, J.B. and Sheldon, M.G., (1985). Clinical Decision = Patient with Problem + Doctor with Problem. This volume.

Howie, J.G.R. (1985). The consultation - a multi-purpose framework. This volume.

Hull, FM. (1985) : The Consultation Process. This volume.

6
Discussion of the Papers by McWhinney and Levenstein

David Pendleton

As a behavioural scientist, I approached the two papers having in mind the decision-making literature from my own discipline. If I set out the basics of this literature, my subsequent comments will become more intelligible.

Decision-making implies making choices amongst alternatives but everything on which the choice is based is essentially subjective. The front running theory of decision-making in social psychology is based on the individual's values and expectations. The model is proposed in which an individual's behaviour is based on intentions. These intentions, in turn, are based on the individual's desire for certain outcomes and his/her estimate of how likely each outcome is. Figure 1 shows these relationships (Sutton 1979).

Naturally enough, as we see the effects of our behaviour we learn to modify our expectations, but our values change much more slowly. Thus our aims and our expectations influence our behaviour. But the insistence on the subjectivity of all of this carries an important consequence, namely, that we cannot understand anyone's behaviour unless we know his/her view of the alternatives. We need to know the range of possibilities conceived, the desirability of the outcomes of each alternative and how likely the outcomes are seen to be.

Subjective Expected Utility Theory

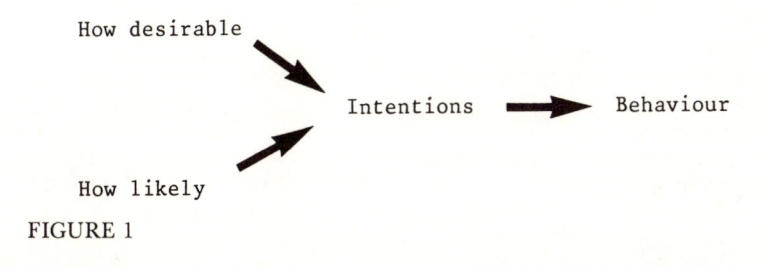

How desirable → Intentions → Behaviour
How likely ↗

FIGURE 1

The papers by McWhinney and by Levenstein articulated the settings in which decisions are made. Levenstein described the consultation - the location for the decision-making. McWhinney described the doctor's orientation to medical practice - the psychological context for the decision-making. Neither chose to write about decision-making per se. In order to write about decision-making the authors would have had to have set out the doctor's definition of his/her own legitimate work, his aims, his range of perceived alternatives, the weighting of the outcomes of the alternatives (how desirable or consistent with the aims) and the doctor's own estimate of achieving the perceived outcomes (how likely to be successful). It is only in this context that intentional behaviour makes sense. The doctor-versus patient-centred debate is at the most general level. Decision-making is a much lower level activity than the level of this distinction though decisions will be influenced by the doctor's orientation. Thus McWhinney's paper may have an unhelpful title but extremely helpful content.

Levenstein's model for the consultation is a welcome attempt on a clinician's part to make explicit the principles according to which he practices and teaches. We all have models of this kind but not all clinicians are sufficiently aware of their models to describe them.

In the introduction to Levenstein's paper, much is said to have been "accepted". A notable example of this is that general practice uses a patient-centred model. Unfortunately, this may be more a feature of the evolving rhetoric of general practice than a reflection of practice per se. The work of Cartwright and Anderson (1981) and of Tuckett (1982) show us only too well that what is practised is usually doctor-centred medicine. The rhetoric has rather left practice behind but general practice is evolving.

There are two strong language sets in general practice. There is the language set of "the surgery" and the set of "the consultation". In the former are ideas such as control, clear instructions and explanations, compliance, reassurance and patient education. The implications are of an active doctor and a passive recipient of care. Indeed, the very word "patient" may be part of this language set. Ideas which surround the idea of "the consultation" would include shared decisions, exchange of views, agreed plans, mutual support and understanding. The rather different implication here is of a negotiation between equals.

The history of general practice can be cast as a journey from the surgery to the consultation.

In the 1950's and the 1960's the first landmark was passed when Michael Balint taught that doctors and patients are alike in that they each have feelings in the consultation which influence their behaviour. In the 1960's and 1970's the concept of Health Beliefs was introduced and applied in many studies to patients. But the implication that some may have drawn is that, whereas patients have mere beliefs, doctors have medical knowledge. Here the physician may need to be reminded that he/she has values, attitudes and beliefs too which influence his/her decision-making and behaviour. Further, "medical knowledge" changes with considerable speed and is interpreted by each individual physician. Thus the doctors belief system and intentions need to be investigated with some urgency.

This will be the second landmark and will enable us to recognise that a consultation is a meeting of two people - each trying to understand what is happening, each with an agenda and each with theories about health and illness. Rationality is not the exclusive province of either participant - it is the information base which is most different.

REFERENCES

Cartwright, A. and Anderson, R. (1981) General Practice Revisited, London, Tavistock.

Sutton, S. (1979) Can subjective expected utility theory explain smokers' decisions to try to stop smoking? In Oborne, D. et al (eds.) Research in Psychology and Medicine Vol II. London, Academic Press.

Tuckett, D. (1982) Final report on the patient project. London, Health Education Council.

7
Diagnosis: Process not Product

Janet Gale and Philip Marsden

In this paper we hope to show that diagnosis can most usefully be seen as a process of thinking rather than a product of clinical enquiry. In doing so, it will be necessary to put our work in context by considering the variety of ways in which diagnosis, as process or product, has been conceptualised and presented by other workers and the assumptions, limitations and implications which are inherent in those ways. Our own research into the process of diagnosis has concentrated on final year medical students, house officers and registrars in general (hospital) medicine. Thus it is necessary for us to establish the generalisability of our findings to the general practice context. The presentation of our results will include a brief description of our research methodology to establish the validity of our data since unsubstantiated, speculative assertions are often made about the nature of the clinician's thinking process. The description of our findings includes particularly a discussion of change and development within the individual clinician which bears upon the hospital training - general practice transition as well as the learning effects of clinical practice itself.

1) WHAT IS DIAGNOSIS? PROCESS NOT PRODUCT

The term 'diagnosis' can be used to imply a finite and definitive stage to be achieved during patient care and to indicate a fairly narrow sample of the clinician's necessary repertoire, not taking into account the wide range of factors, variables, aspects, skills and behaviours which make up the clinical consultation. If we take the term 'diagnosis' simply to mean all of the items appearing in the WHO International Classification of Disease, as quoted in "The Future General Practitioner" (1972), then such implications would be upheld. However, in this paper we do not use the word 'diagnosis' in this way. For us, the term encompasses those processes whereby the clinician interprets clinical information, follows and chooses among his thoughts about what is wrong with the patient in any given set of circumstances. Clearly, those processes occur in close association with a variety of interpersonal skills and techniques for collecting information (RCGP, 1972). However, for analytical purposes, such phenomena, although crucial to the success of the consultation, can be separated off from the central thinking of the clinician directed at discovering what, if anything, is the problem and what, if anything, is to be done about it during or after its identification. Our definition of diagnosis is concerned only with this aspect of the consultation, with the doctor's cognitive or thinking processes.

Having said this, it is necessary to clarify and resolve one important issue for general practice. That issue concerns the debate which focusses on the relationship between 'diagnosis' and 'management'. Brooke & Sheldon (this publication) point out that there is evidence that the focus of general practice decisions is in management rather than diagnosis, while McWhinney (1980) argues that the conventional 'diagnosis' merely defines the point at which management decisions can be taken. This echoes Cohen's (1943) definition of diagnosis (quoted by Howie, 1972) as a "provisional formula designed for action" and Crombie's (1963) analogy of diagnoses as "stepping stones" to problem management. "The Future General Practitioner" (RCGP, 1972) is more precise:

> "The diagnosis is a crucial achievement which opens the way to prognosis and treatment .... (But it) must still be regarded as previsional, until supported by the subsequent course of the case or the response to specific treatment".

Nevertheless, "on the basis of (diagnoses) doctors can propose and implement solutions". We are beginning to see, then, that even the static definition of diagnosis as a product or an entity has distinct elements of process included in it. Diagnosis, on either definition, and management are inextricably linked. Using the static 'product' definition, the one (diagnosis) precedes the other; while using the process definition, the one (diagnostic process) subsumes the other (management). This latter view is supported by our own findings (see Section 4 ii below) in that the diagnostic thinking process is nowhere characterised by an unalterable end point. We would regard management decisions as an integral part of the diagnostic process and not as an alternative formulation or focus. This being so, management action can be taken before anything approaching the International Classification of Disease 'diagnosis' is achieved. Symptoms or signs alone often prompt management action. For example,

> "I don't know what is wrong but I know he is ill. Please admit".

> "Dialyse first - diagnose second"

> "Whatever else is wrong he is clearly resentful. I must modify my approach to get anywhere near his problem".

"With that sort of history I would just give antacids and see if it cleared up rather than take things further now"

Since cases such as this can and do occur, our own description of the diagnostic thinking process does not include the unqualified term 'diagnosis', and does not imply that management action is a subsequent event; it is part of the process.

2) WAYS OF CONCEPTUALISING THE DIAGNOSTIC PROCESS

The title of this symposium is "Decision-Making in General Practice". That fact alone renders this section of our paper necessary, for the term "decision-making" implies assumptions, directions and limitations with which our own contribution might not comply. In other words, to have selected the term "decision-making" already tends to channel and limit ways of discussing what the general practitioner does and how he/she might be aided in doing it. This would be so for whatever term is selected. Table 1 illustrates some of the variety of terms used.

Given such a variety, it is crucial to mutual understanding and progress that the derivations and implications of each term are made explicit so that the theoretical orientation, purpose and intentions of each author are quite clear. We then can achieve a rational basis for assessing, comparing and using the variety of approaches.

Each of the terms shown in Table 1 implies, either consciously or unconsciously, a certain model of thinking and most come from easily identifiable schools of thought in psychology. So when a writer or researcher uses these terms, his/her possible ways of looking at or explaining what doctors do are limited. He/she has made prior assumptions about the likely explanation. It is as though a certain neurological disease were called 'viral multiple sclerosis'. The name of the disease would be a most powerful constraint on the development of other explanations of the disease process. We begin to think differently about the original, as a result of the words we use to describe it. And so it is with doctors' thinking.

In this way 'problem-solving' implies the view of human thinking which information processing theories expound; 'reasoning' and 'inference' imply some formal logical process; 'judgement' implies some cognitive weighing and balancing; 'decision-making' implies other forms of logical thinking based on formal quantitative or algebraic decision models. From this it is clear that, although the researchers who use all these different terms might be looking at the same phenomenon (doctors or students trying to find out what is wrong with patients), they have chosen to use different frames of reference to describe it. Different explanations of the same phenomenon arise for a number of reasons. There seem to be two powerful ones. Firstly, different researchers themselves have different theoretical

TERMINOLOGY/DESCRIPTION	AUTHORS	DATE
Diagnostic process	Dudley	1969
Diagnosis as cognitive skill	Taylor et al	1971
Clinical judgment	Feinstein Schwarz et al Meals Elstein	1967 1973 1973 1976
Diagnostic reasoning	Sprafka & Elstein	1974
Medical judgment	Knafl & Burkett	1975
Decision making	McWhinney Murray et al Mayou Brooke	1972, 1980 1977 1978 (this publication)
Clinical inference/logical/ scientific method	Medawar Dudley Forstrom	1969 1970, 1982 1977
Problem solving	Barrows & Bennett Brooke Cutler	1972 (this publication) 1979
Clinical cognition	Pauker et al	1976
Medical problem solving Clinical reasoning Medical thinking	Elstein et al	1978
Clinical reasoning process	Barrows & Tamblyn	1980
Diagnostic thinking process	Gale Gale & Marsden	1982 1983
Clinical problem solving process	Gale & Marsden	1982
Pattern recognition	Style Scadding Barrows et al	1979 1967 1978
Intuition	Style	1979

TABLE 1: TERMINOLOGY USED TO DESCRIBE STUDENTS' AND DOCTORS' THINKING

orientations, different knowledge bases and feel more or less familiar and happy with different kinds of explanation. "Pattern recognition" is just such an explanation, put forward by a number of people (Scadding, 1976; Hamilton, 1966; Gorry, 1970; Ridderikhoff, 1982; RCGP, 1972). It seems to make sense; the term seems understandable; the clinician could see the results of his thinking in such a way. However, it is both inaccurate and inadequate as an explanation obscuring a variety of complex cognitive processes which result in that "recognition" (Gale, 1980), yet use of the term limits other explanations. Secondly, researchers have different purposes for undertaking their work, and different kinds of explanation may well be satisfactory for different kinds of purpose. Let us consider, firstly, the effects of different theoretical orientations on the outcome of research into doctors' and students' thinking.

Clearly, a major determinant of research outcome is research methods. Thus if, like Kleinmuntz (1968) or Schwarz et al (1973), a researcher asks a clinician to work his way through a decision tree, the resultant model of the clinician's thinking will be related to some kind of decision theory. It may well be that, as Schwarz et al (1973) suggest, "most physicians will find the diagrammatic representation . . . quite in keeping with their thinking about medical problems", but it still is just a diagrammatic representation, and not an accurate description of cognition.

Similar arguments would apply to statistical, computer-based and probabilistic models. But Habbema and van der Maas (1981) point out that "statistical decision theory is a normative or prescriptive approach to medical decision-making. It describes how decisions should be made. It is in contrast with descriptive models which tell us how decisions are made". We might not agree with Habbema and van der Maas that decisions should be made in this way or that, but the point they make is valid and important. Thus statistical, algebraic and decision theories are paramorphic (ie. symbolic) representations of the doctor's thinking, not isomorphic (ie. exact replication) ones. In order to attain a description rather than symbolic representation of such thinking, we must consider work which takes a study of the clinician as its major reference point, and descriptive cognitive psychology as its theoretical and methodological basis. Our own approach is in this line.

As well as various theoretical orientations, workers also have different purposes. Such purposes are diverse and include attempts to systematise, to model, to enhance and to describe thinking processes. They also include intentions to alter or add to the doctor's thinking by adding another dimension.

There is little doubt that by adopting a system of numerical weighting of clinical features using some method such as score cards with a decision system, resultant benefits such as a reduction in hospital referral may be calculated to accrue (Knill-Jones, 1977).

Symptoms and signs can be identified which discriminate between important (but defined) entities such as acute appendicitis and non-specific abdominal pain (Neutra, 1977) and much other work testifies to the ability of discriminant analysis to improve efficienty of investigation (Keighley et al, 1976). Such approaches including those using Bayes' theorem (Knill-Jones, 1975) have had as their immediate goal the improvement of medical practice by improving the doctor's choice and use of information. They also suggest new tools, such as computers, to help the clinician combine the information available. What they do not do in any way is to describe what the clinician, faced with a real patient, actually does. However, it is well recognised that such aids to the diagnostic process cannot be integrated into clinical practice successfully unless the actual thinking processes of the clinician are known and understood (Ridderikhoff, this publication; Brooke et al 1983). We may now proceed to consideration of whether that process and understanding are the same in hospital and general practice settings, since our own research was conducted in medical schools and hospitals and we now intend to apply it to general practice.

3) THE DIAGNOSTIC PROCESS AND GENERAL PRACTICE

Unquestionably, there are profound and significant differences between hospital practice and general practice. The issue for us, however, concerns whether or not these differences are located within or affect the diagnostic thinking processes of the clinicians concerned. The major differences identified can be summarised as follows:

In terms of clinical content, a general practitioner would tend to see a wider range of problems presenting at an earlier stage than a hospital specialist (Brooke et al, 1983) and those problems might often be seen as "illness" (ie. "the patient's total experience of being unwell") whereas in hospital medicine the clinician may well focus more sharply on the "disease" (ie. "a pathological process of the body or the mind") (RCGP, 1972). The general practitioner might also often have to address questions which rarely appear in hospital practice, such as "Who should be the patient?" and "Who should be the doctor?" (RCGP, 1972). The wide range and nature of problems and questions in general practice might also mean that the general practitioner more "often has to make decisions without the necessary knowledge to hand" (Brooke et al, 1984). As a corollary, he/she might also have different aims from those of the specialist and be more likely to concentrate on "eliminative diagnosis" (Crombie, 1963) or splitting patients into large binary groups than achieving "exact histological diagnosis" (Brooke et al 1984). It is possible, however, that hospital doctors might question the myth of the specialist's affinity for definitive diagnosis.

Patients in hospital are often more seriously ill than those seen in general practice so the incidence of "death or cure" with the attendant revelations of post mortem examination and proof by therapeutic outcome is higher. Hospital doctors have access to many tests and diagnostic procedures which also tend to raise the "definitely diagnosed" rate. It is very often the case, however, that such tests merely have the effect of shortening the period of uncertainty. During the actual process of assessment there is considerable diagnostic doubt. It lasts for a shorter period but nevertheless antibiotics are still given before chest x-rays are obtained, multiple treatment without firm diagnosis often occurs in acute situations and the "definitive diagnosis" of the discharge summary is often merely an abstraction obtained retrospectively. The myth of the faultless hospital assessment also is perpetuated by the long established education and "audit" procedures of the hospital, the grand round, case presentation, or CPC in which clinical reality is often remodelled into a smoother, more logical and more satisfactory version. In point of fact, our own research shows that the final, unalterable "diagnosis" is not a feature of hospital doctors' thinking while assessing a clinical situation.

In terms of organisation, it appears that general practice has a different, more extended time-scale from that of hospital medicine, (RCGP, 1972), clinical encounters in general practice occurring as a series over a period of time (Bentsen, this publication), "single frames in a long-running cine file", (Howie, this publication).

Such differences of content and organisation as these do not seem to be influential when considering the clinician's thinking processes or models thereof. Indeed, the thinking of both hospital doctors and general practitioners has been subject to the same descriptions and representations as pattern recognition (Scadding, 1967; RCGP, 1972), as hypothesis generation and testing (Barrows et al, 1982; Style, 1979), as probabilistic or predictive (McWhinney, 1980; Taylor et al, 1971). Indeed, Barrows et al (1982) in a rare empirical study show that general practitioners and hospital doctors use the same "multiple hypothesis-guided, problem orientated enquiry". The only differences discovered showed, predictably, that the general practitioners asked fewer questions and spent less time with the patient, than did hospital specialists. Given this discussion, then, it is difficult to disagree with Bentsen (1980) that "the difference between generalist and specialist practice is one of quantities rather than quality" or with the RCGP (1972) that "the method which the specialist uses in the hospital out-patient department, and which the general practitioner employs in his consulting room, is identical". On this basis we can move on to describe our own research and findings in the firm belief that, although based on hospital practice, they apply equally to the general practitioner.

4) THE PROCESS OF DIAGNOSIS

The aim of our research was to describe the actual cognitive or thinking processes of the clinician, not to build a model of these, but to describe in psychological terms exactly what goes on inside the clinician's head. A number of workers have already shown that clinicians use a process of hypothesis generation and testing (Elstein et al. 1978; Barrows and Tamblyn, 1980), but such a process is characteristic of all adult thinking (Inhelder and Piaget, 1958) and does not describe the specific thinking processes or cognitive mechanisms involved in the clinician actually forming an hypothesis, testing it, and making a decision about what is wrong or what to do. We also considered that a more precise description of the clinician's thinking processes would, by definition, be more accurate and so more helpful in developing pedagogical strategies, tracing and explaining the development from neophyte to expert, research into which had shown a confused and contradictory picture (Gale, 1980), and in helping individuals to analyse their own practice.

(i) Methodology

Details and discussion of rationale, reliability, validity and statistical analyses are available in Gale (1980) and Gale and Marsden (1983).

The subjects of the study were 22 final year clinical medical students, 22 pre-registration house officers and 22 post-MRCP registrars with a mean of 5.2 years of clinical practice. All subjects trained at traditional medical schools. Each subject conducted a clinical interview with a real patient. The interview was videorecorded. Immediately following the completion of the clinical interview, the subject and researcher reviewed the videotape in short sections between which the subject commented in detail on his or her own underlying thoughts as they had occurred while interviewing the patient. After audio recording and transcription, these data were subjected to rigorous content analysis to reveal the specific thinking processes involved.

(ii) Results: The Diagnostic Thinking Process

Content analysis of data and reference to the psychological literature yielded a detailed description and explanation of the diagnostic thinking process which is presented in Table 2 and can be summarised in the following points, each of which is accompanied by an illustrated example. These points reflect the 'psychological factors' identified in Table 2.

1. An individual's perception of a diagnostic problem is dependent upon the way that person's knowledge is structured or organised in his/her memory. Not only might people have different knowledge, but the same knowledge can be structured in memory in different ways by different people.

EXAMPLE 1

MEMORY STRUCTURE OF CLINICIAN A	MEMORY STRUCTURE OF CLINICIAN B
Tremor only with warm hands Myopathy Absence of tachycardia is against Goitre with bruit	Tremor Tachycardia Exophthalmos Warm hands Goitre

The two boxes illustrate diagrammatically part of the possible memory structures for physical signs of thyrotoxicosis of two clinicians. Comparison of the boxes shows that not only do these two people have different knowledge but also that similar knowledge can be organised in different ways.

2. At no point in the clinical interview does the clinician gather any information without responding to or evaluating it immediately either by interpreting it in some way or by judging it to be uninterpretable to him/her without further enquiry. These responses are related to the individual's own memory structures and their means of access.

EXAMPLE 2

When a group of seven medical students was told at the beginning of a clinical interview that a 22 year old female patient was complaining of pain in the legs, breathlessness and feeling distant, their immediate individual responses were as follows:

"Deep vein thrombosis" (x2)
"Anxiety"
"I want to know what she means by feeling distant"
"DVT with pulmonary embolus"
"How long has she had trouble?"
"I'd want to know more".

Each student made some active response to the initial information. Passive receipt of information without mentally reacting to it in some way did not occur. The students' responses were either interpretative or were judgements not to interpret without further enquiry. This variety of responses occurred because the students had a variety of individual memory structures, though clearly there are also broad similarities. However, this group of students also demonstrated that memory structures can be present but not used. So when told that the patient had been found to be suffering from emotional hyperventilation, this enabled the students to use their own knowledge of this subject previously not accessed. The majority could explain all the clinical features pathophysiologically; two had heard of 'distant feelings' in this condition and one student had actually suffered from the condition. Despite having appropriate knowledge this had not been 'accessed' in the clinical context.

3. The link between knowledge structures in memory and a given clinical situation is formed by specially significant items of information ('forceful features'). These 'neon-light items' are not a property of the clinical information itself, but are subjectively derived by the individual from experience and constitute part of that person's memory structure.

EXAMPLE 3

The following diagram shows an array of clinical information. Three clinicians, when presented with this array, made three different interpretations of it because different pieces of information 'seemed to strike' them as important. Thus each clinician had identified different forceful features from among the array, because in each clinician different pieces of clinical information assumed greatest importance. The diagram shows which pieces of information acted as forceful features in relation to each different interpretation made

CLINICIAN'S INTERPRETATIONS	LINKS TO FORCEFUL FEATURES	CLINICAL INFORMATION ARRAY

- WOMAN OF 51
- 2 YEAR HISTORY OF DIARRHOEA AFTER EATING
- ATTACKS OF SHAKING OF HANDS
- PUERPERAL DEPRESSION AFTER SECOND CHILD
- GASTRIC ULCER TREATED SURGICALLY 5 YEARS AGO
- FAMILY HISTORY (MOTHER, SISTER) OF THYROTOXICOSIS

1. Thyrotoxicosis
2. Dumping syndrome
3. Psychiatric

Forceful features act as 'keys' to memory, providing the mechanism for gaining access to the information stored there. What acts as a forceful feature depends on the way the person has organised his/her knowledge in the memory store. As Example 2, above, shows, relevant information might be stored in a clinician's memory, but if it is not organised such that it is accessible via forceful features that are clinically relevant, it will not be of use when appropriate.

Note As Example 3 shows, a forceful feature can be made up of any number of pieces of information. Equally, the same forceful feature can be the 'key' to many memory structures.

4. Once an interpretation has been made, it causes the clinician to expect or search for further information in a manner determined by his/her individual memory structures.

EXAMPLE 4

Gale and Marsden (1983) quote part of an interview with a student who was explaining why he had followed a certain line of questioning with a patient. The student explains:

"You always expect other symptoms. If he's got a cardiac complaint like that, especially coming on for no apparent reason, you have to think of pain or anything else or whether he felt dizzy, fainted, nausea, anything which may be associated with his chest complaint. In fact, I found out that he did have dizzy spells so I pursued that a bit further."

So, because information is stored in memory in organised, structured ways, one piece of information leads the clinician to wonder about related pieces of information and question the patient accordingly. This student's interpretation of "a cardiac complaint" caused him to ask a series of related questions and elicit new information.

---

5. As the interview proceeds, reinterpretation of the clinical information occurs by a process of relating it to different memory structures.

EXAMPLE 5

Example 3, above, has demonstrated the forceful feature. We can now consider how forceful features come into play to enable (or force) the clinician to make new interpretations. Consider the following example in which a clinician, when initially presented with a patient complaining of headache and vomiting, used these as a forceful feature and extrapolated to an interpretation of migraine. On reflection, he used the same information to make the different interpretation of febrile headache. He thus reinterpreted the same information. When he then discovered that the patient had a pulse rate of 60 per minute, he used all three pieces of information to make a new interpretation of raised intracranial pressure. He thus reinterpreted in the presence of new information. Now we can see two forms of reinterpretation: firstly, reinterpretation of the same information by relating it to different memory structures; secondly, reinterpreting in the presence of new information which yields a new forceful feature and so opens the door to a different memory structure and a new interpretation

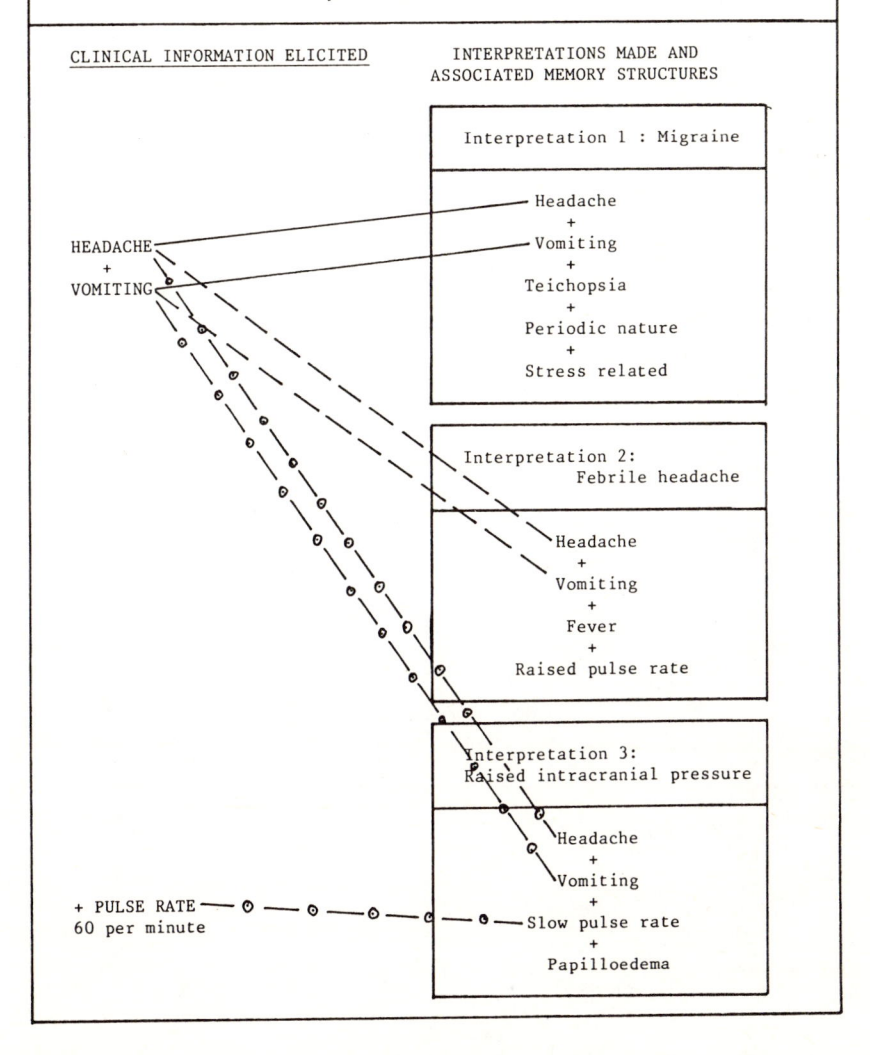

CLINICAL INFORMATION ELICITED   INTERPRETATIONS MADE AND ASSOCIATED MEMORY STRUCTURES

HEADACHE
+
VOMITING

Interpretation 1 : Migraine

Headache
+
Vomiting
+
Teichopsia
+
Periodic nature
+
Stress related

Interpretation 2:
Febrile headache

Headache
+
Vomiting
+
Fever
+
Raised pulse rate

Interpretation 3:
Raised intracranial pressure

Headache
+
Vomiting
+
Slow pulse rate
+
Papilloedema

+ PULSE RATE
60 per minute

EXAMPLE 6

Below are given extracts from three interviews with a patient, each by a different clinician.

The patient is a woman of 63 who has been admitted to hospital after feeling faint and then losing consciousness in the bathroom. The patient suffers from angina which is occasional and not usually severe but she has recently developed recurrent paroxysmal supra-ventricular tachycardia which on this occasion was followed by severe chest pain and myocardial infarction.

CLINICIAN 1	PATIENT	COMMENT
When you felt faint did you get any tightness in the chest?	In my chest and throat I thought "It's just the anxiety coming back". I couldn't breathe.	The subsequent course of the interview follows on from information given by the patient.
Have you had it before, this tightness?	Yes, the anxiety, but this time it didn't go away.	
How long have you had anxiety?	Since I was a child.	

CLINICIAN 2		
How many pillows do you use? Do you wake up short of breath?	Three here. Two at home. No, but I sometimes get this rapid heart beat.	The clinician determines the course of the interview by continuing to pursue his own pre-existing interpretation of left ventricular failure. Some highly relevant information from the patient is here passed by to be returned to later.
But do you get a cough with phlegm? Is there blood in it?	Yes, I get a lot of phlegm. No.	

CLINICIAN 3		
Have you had tightness in the chest before on exercise or when you are nervous	Mainly after climbing stairs.	The subsequent course of the interview is determined by a question derived from a category of the routine history.
What do you do?	Rest	
How long does it take to go?	About a minute.	
Fine. How are your waterworks?	Well, I take a water tablet, but all right.	

6. At any point in the interview the clinician's next enquiry might occur as a result of either new information from the patient or the clinician's pre-existing interpretations or a category of the routine history.

7. At the end of the interview the clinician treats each interpretation as either confirmed or eliminated or not proven either way. Such judgements are potentially changeable.

EXAMPLE 7

Gale and Marsden (1983) report a variety of explanations given by students, house officers and clinicians of their conclusions about their patients' diagnoses after a clinical interview. Clinicians demonstrate three main ways of dealing with their interpretations. These are discussed further below as Processes 12, 13 and 14 but are named here in the left hand column, while the right hand column reports associated illustrative statements made by clinicians:

FATE OF INTERPRETATIONS	CLINICIANS ILLUSTRATIVE STATEMENTS
Confirmation of an interpretation	"I'm convinced by now that it's diagnosis X."
	"He's describing syndrome X which is A plus B plus C due to E."
Elimination of an interpretation	"I'd pretty well dismissed diagnosis X because he hadn't got symptom Y."
	"I asked about X because it can cause diagnosis Y, but she hadn't got X."
Postponement of judgment about an interpretation	"I'd put my money on diagnosis X if I had to but I couldn't really say with a great deal of certainty that that's what happened to her."
	"She's the right category for disease X but I don't know any questions that could diagnose that."

It is important to note that any of these statements could be seen as interim, as the best possible statement at the time. Each could be altered or reviewed by subsequent clinical events or by the clinician's own reinterpretation of the existing clinical information, as shown in Example 5.

8. Diagnostic errors occur as a result of inadequacy, inappropriateness or inaccessibility of memory structures, or of failure to use an appropriate range of thinking processes, or clinging to an incorrect interpretation (set effect).

EXAMPLE 8

Gale and Marsden (1983) give a variety of examples from their research studies of mechanisms of error in the diagnostic thinking processes of students, house officers and registrars. They stress, however, that:
". . . the errors to be discussed are not systematic and often are rare . . . (and) although the errors discussed were identified in the sample of subjects., in many cases they were also rectified during the course of the interview."

The following explanatory comments of some of the subjects of the study exemplify some main mechanisms of error:

MECHANISM OF ERROR	CLINICIANS' ILLUSTRATIVE STATEMENTS
Inadequate memory structure	"Symptoms kept cropping up all over the place that I hadn't thought to ask about."
	". . . but the deafness; I'm not a neurologist; I can't remember what's nerve deafness and what's bone deafness. I just discarded it straight away."
Inappropriate memory structure	"I know that you get churning bowel sounds and borborygmi in obstruction but it just didn't seem important to me at the time."
	"Watery eyes are at the bottom of my list for myxoedema."
Failure to use an appropriate range of thinking processes	"I just dropped it, I didn't follow it up."
Set effect (clinging to an incorrect interpretation	One clinician's patient had Crohn's disease. He complained of stomach pains not affected by food and diarrhoea with blood in it. The doctor was 'set' towards an interpretation of functional diarrhoea. At one point he responded as follows: "I think this is functional because pain can accompany it, but blood should not. The blood could be haemorrhoids." The patient then told of nocturnal diarrhoea but the clinician clung to his 'set': "Not usual with functional diarrhoea but it could mean he started off with that and has developed something else." This clinician continued to defend his 'set' interpretation against all contrary evidence, and never reached the correct diagnosis.

Diagnosis: Process not Product

9. No statistically significant differences were found in the range of 14 thinking processes (see below) available to students and experienced clinicians. Superior diagnostic performance can best be attributed to differences in memory structure and their accessibility.

EXAMPLE 9

The following example shows that an inexperienced (student) clinician and an experienced (registrar) clinician use the same thinking processes, while the content of their thoughts is different. The example is a real one, although the responses have been selected to illustrate the point clearly that clinicians at all levels think in the same ways and that experience and expertise are not related to the development of new ways of thinking, but rather are a function of developing increasingly appropriate and usable memory structures of knowledge.

CLINICAL INFORMATION
A 63 YEAR OLD MAN WHO COMPLAINED OF A BLACKOUT IN THE TOILET.

STUDENT'S RESPONSE: ? Angina   REGISTRAR'S RESPONSE: ? Micturition syncope

COMMENT

Thought content — The student interpreted this history as 'angina' despite lack of any history of chest pains. He found that "blackout" made him think only of angina. The registrar made a very different interpretation based on "blackout in the toilet" which was more appropriate.

Thought process — Both student and registrar recognised a forceful feature (albeit different ones) and accessed a memory structure, one inappropriate (angina), one appropriate (micturition syncope).

STUDENT'S SUBSEQUENT QUESTION   REGISTRAR'S SUBSEQUENT QUESTIONS:
Have you had any heart trouble?   Did you completely black out?
                                        Was there any warning?
                                        Were you standing at the time?
                                        Were you straining to pass water at the time?
                                        Has this happened before?

COMMENT

Thought content — The student could find only one question to ask, which was inappropriate to the extent that it would neither confirm nor rule out angina. The registrar had available a series of tightly organised, highly appropriate questions which reflect a relevant, well-structured memory which is clearly more elaborated than that of the student who was at the beginning of his clinical course.

Thought process — Both student and registrar followed up their interpretation by questioning. Both did this by formulating questions working from their accessed memory structures related to the interpretations they had made.

STAGE	THINKING PROCESS	PSYCHOLOGICAL FACTORS
I INITIATION	1. Pre-diagnostic interpretation 2. Diagnostic interpretation 3. Judgment of need for further enquiry	Instantaneous response always active Structure of memory Forceful feature
II PROGRESS	4. Expecting, searching for specific information 5. Reinterpretation: no new information 6. Reinterpretation: with new information	Assessment of interpretations Reinterpretation - shift of force - multiple interpretations Restructuring
	7. Enquiry responsive to elicited information 8. Enquiry responsive to clinician's interpretations 9. Routine enquiry	Enquiry pattern subject to variety of influences
	10. Failure to make specific enquiry 11. Failure to make general enquiry	Enquiry failures Problems in 'thinking' on one's feet
III RESOLUTION	12. Active confirmation of an interpretation 13. Active elimination of an interpretation 14. Postponement of judgment	Reversible judgment Psychological probability
ANY STAGE		Set effect (clinging to a favoured interpretation). Use of non-standard information. Designation of irrelevance of information. Failure to make correct interpretations.

TABLE 2: SUMMARY OF THE DIAGNOSTIC THINKING PROCESS, ITS STAGES AND UNDERLYING PSYCHOLOGICAL FACTORS

Table 2 shows that within this overall description summarised in nine points and examples, 14 specific thinking processes were identified. These represent a range upon which the clinician can draw in any one instance. We would not necessarily expect all thinking processes to be called into service on all occasions by all clinicians. Neither would we necessarily expect them all to be used appropriately on all occasions. Cognitive errors do occur. These 14 processes are simply the range which students and clinicians have at their command. The thinking processes which are named in Table 2 can be described and exemplified as follows:

PROCESS 1 Pre-diagnostic interpretation of clinical information

    Definition An active interpretation of the clinical information available where the result of this activity is not sufficiently specific to constitute a possible diagnosis.

    Examples
(i) The interpretation may be at a relatively undefined level:

    eg. "Something wrong with . . ."

    "Myocardial problem"

(ii) The interpretation may be at a relatively defined level:

    eg. "A metabolic abnormality"

    "Anaemia caused by blood loss"

PROCESS 2 Diagnostic interpretation of clinical information

    Definition An active interpretation of clinical information where a pathophysiological process is indicated with a degree of specificity which is sufficient for a diagnosis.

    Examples
(i) "Carcinoma of the pancreas"

(ii) "Acromegaly"

PROCESS 3	Judgment of need for further general or clarifying enquiry not stemming from either pre-diagnostic or diagnostic interpretations
Definition	Where the clinician enquires further about the patient's symptoms, signs, etc. for clarification or seeks to clarify the patient's statement.
Examples	(i) "I was asking how the pain affected him."
	(ii) "I asked her how she didn't feel well."
PROCESS 4	Expecting, searching for or planning to search for specific features (symptoms, signs, tests, etc.) of disease or treatment of disease
Definition	Where the clinician shows expectation of certain clinical information or considers certain features of disease likely or possible in the patient, given the information already elicited.
Examples	(i) "If we investigated the patient, I'd imagine we'd find X."
	(ii) "I'm asking these questions because the patient may have X as part of her syndrome."
PROCESS 5	Reinterpretation of clinical information, when no new information has been added
Definition	Where an array of clinical information which has already been interpreted in some way becomes amenable to a new interpretation because of a change in the clinician's own thinking and not because new information has been added to the array.
Examples	(i) "It was creeping into my mind/struck me/flashed through my mind that he may have diagnosis X" (when no new information has prompted this).
	(ii) "I suddenly saw that symptoms X and Y were related/separate."

Diagnosis: Process not Product

PROCESS 6   Reinterpretation of clinical information arising from the addition of new information

  Definition   Where an array of clinical information which has already been interpreted in some way becomes amenable to new interpretation because of the addition of new information to the array.

  Examples
- (i) "Symptom X now suggests that it may be diagnosis Y."
- (ii) "I'd thought of diagnosis X, but when I asked further questions, I realised that diagnosis Y was the case."

PROCESS 7   Enquiry responsive to elicited information

  Definition   Where the course of the interview as directed by the clinician is determined by, or follows on from, the flow of information as presented by the patient.

  Examples
- (i) Not where the clinician merely allows the patient to talk without interruption.
- (ii) Not where the clinician merely seeks clarification or elaboration of information given to the patient.
- (iii) "If a system came up, I dealt with it there instead of waiting for the systematic enquiry."
- (iv) "I decided to do the CVS there because it was relevant to what she just mentioned."

PROCESS 8   Enquiry determined by the clinician's interpretations

  Definition   Where the course of the interview is determined by the clinician's requirement actively to test his/her interpretations of the clinical information.

  Examples
- (i) "I was thinking in terms of diagnosis X, so I asked about symptom X."
- (ii) "I was looking for symptoms X, Y and Z."

PROCESS 9 — Routine enquiry

Definition — Where the clinician conducts, or attempts to conduct, the interview according to a routine format as defined by the standard clinical history, defined as follows:

1. Presenting complaint.

2. History of the present complaint.

3. Symptomatic survey (by systems):

    (a) Cardiovascular

    (b) Respiratory

    (c) Locomotor

    (d) Genito-urinary

    (e) Gastro-intestinal

    (f) Neurological

    (g) General

4. Past medical history.

5. Family history.

6. Social history.

7. Drug survey.

Examples

(i) "This is just routine/general enquiry."

(ii) "He (the patient) was getting my systems mucked up, so that had to wait."

PROCESS 10 — Failure to make specific enquiry

Definition — Where the clinician identifies, in retrospect, his/her own failure to make relevant, specific enquiry concerning the patient's problems, symptoms, signs etc.

Examples

(i) "I should have gone into that symptom in more depth, but I forgot."

(ii) "Symptoms kept cropping up all over the place that I hadn't thought to ask about."

PROCESS 11		Failure to make general enquiry
Definition		Where the clinician identifies, in retrospect, his/her own failure to make sufficient routine, general or screening enquiry.
Examples	(i)	"This is just a superficial social history, it might be worth pursuing it a bit more".
	(ii)	"I could have asked a lot more questions about this system, but I tend to forget them unless they seem necessary".
Note:		These processes indicate the clinician's failure at the time, not a failure of knowledge generally, but a failure to "think in action".

PROCESS 12		Active confirmation of an interpretation
Definition		Where the clinician feels that the selected interpretation is confirmed as an actual diagnosis.
Examples	(i)	"My conclusion is that she's suffering from diagnosis X".
	(ii)	"I'm convinced by now that it's diagnosis X".

PROCESS 13		Active elimination of an interpretation*
Definition		Where the clinician eliminates an identified interpretation because of contrary evidence or positive lack of necessary evidence.
		* Passive elimination of interpretation also probably occurs.
Examples	(i)	"I'd pretty well dismissed diagnosis X because he hadn't got symptom Y".
	(ii)	"I'd asked about X because it can cause diagnosis Y, but she hasn't got X".

PROCESS 14   Postponement of judgment

  Definition   Where an identified possible interpretation is neither confirmed nor eliminated by the clinician but is left under postponed judgment.

  Examples   (i)   Where the following are the clinicians' opinions

              (ii)   "It was disease type X, with diagnosis Y high on the list".

                     "She's the right category for disease X, but I don't know any questions that could diagnose that".

Table 2 shows that these 14 processes conveniently can be divided into three stages. This is for analytical purposes only and refers to the career of one interpretation only. It must be emphasised, that these do not refer either to stages in the overall diagnostic thinking process (which will probably be made up of many interpretations) or to temporal points in the clinical interview. The three stages which interpretation goes through we have designated as follows; explanatory examples will be given later:

STAGE 1: Initiation - During this stage the clinician immediately interprets the available clinical information and makes sense of it by imposing some structure or organisation on it by means of recognition of a forceful feature (an item or items of information which are particularly important to him/her which allows access to a particular memory structure).

STAGE 2: Progress - During this stage, the clinician assesses his/her interpretations of the clinical information and might reinterpret it. Restructuring of the clinical array of information occurs either by shift of force involving use of a new forceful feature or by multiple extrapolation to different memory structures from the same forceful feature. History-taking during this stage is determined by a variety of influences identified as Processes 7,8 and 9 above.

STAGE 3: Resolution - At the end of the interview, the clinician treats each interpretation as either confirmed or eliminated or not proven either way. Such judgments are potentially reversible and are made according to subjective judgmental, not objective numerical estimates of probability.

As the clinical interview (spread over any period of time) progresses, the clinician makes many and changing interpretations of the clinical information, and at any point the clinician might be at the stage of initiation of one interpretation, of progress with another, and resolution with yet a third. Example 10 demonstrates this point, showing a doctor considering a patient with breathlessness which in reality was due to asthma. It presents a summary of information elicited and the overlapping stages of initiation, progress and resolution of the doctor's various interpretations.

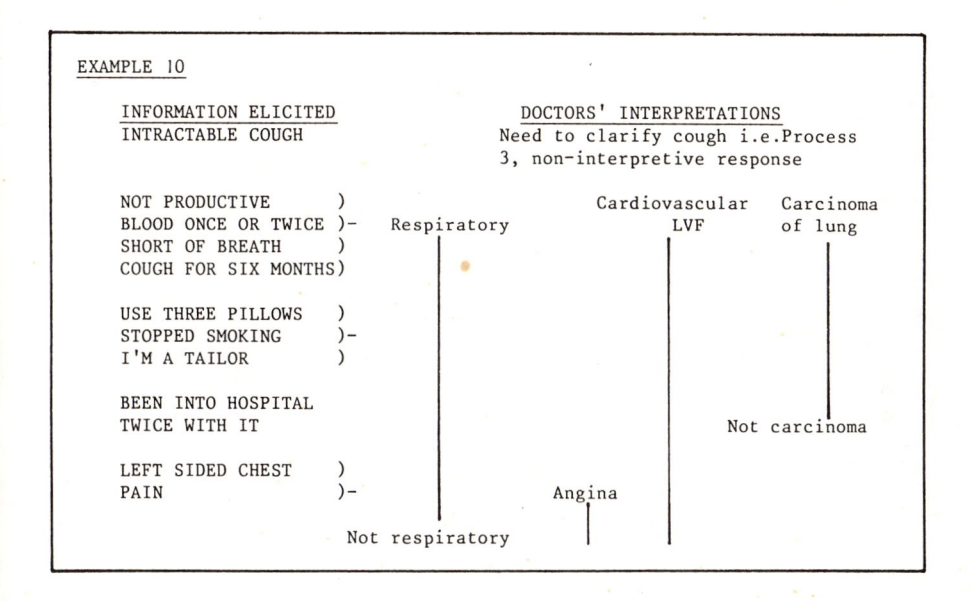

```
EXAMPLE 10

    INFORMATION ELICITED              DOCTORS' INTERPRETATIONS
    INTRACTABLE COUGH                 Need to clarify cough i.e.Process
                                      3, non-interpretive response

    NOT PRODUCTIVE      )                    Cardiovascular    Carcinoma
    BLOOD ONCE OR TWICE )-  Respiratory           LVF          of lung
    SHORT OF BREATH     )
    COUGH FOR SIX MONTHS)

    USE THREE PILLOWS   )
    STOPPED SMOKING     )-
    I'M A TAILOR        )

    BEEN INTO HOSPITAL
    TWICE WITH IT                                              Not carcinoma

    LEFT SIDED CHEST    )
    PAIN                )-
                                         Angina
                     Not respiratory
```

We have presented here a detailed description of the range of thinking processes available to clinicians at all levels of training and experience. However, we would not wish this to be seen as a description of static phenomenon. Experts and experienced clinicians are generally "better" than neophytes. People do develop and learn and adapt as new knowledge and clinical experiences are encountered, or as new practice environments and conditions are entered. The final section of this paper deals with how such changes occur and the implications of this for general practice training and education.

5) CHANGE AND DEVELOPMENT IN THE DIAGNOSTIC THINKING PROCESS: SOME IMPLICATIONS FOR GENERAL PRACTICE

It has already been stated that no statistically significant differences were found in the range of thinking processes available to students, house officers and registrars (Gale and Marsden 1983). These three groups were compared by counting the frequency of pre-diagnostic interpretations of clinical information per person and the frequency of other thinking processes per group. The data were then analysed to determine whether the groups of subjects differed either in the thinking processes they displayed or in the frequency with which they displayed them. A chi-square test revealed no statistically significant difference between groups in relative frequency of pre-diagnostic and diagnostic interpretations of clinical information (chi-square = 1.1581, df = 2, NS). Analysis of variance indicated no statistically significant difference between groups in frequency of the remaining 12 thinking processes (F = 0.3010, df = 2, 63, NS).

It is clear, then, that students, house officers and registrars have available to them the same range of complex diagnostic thinking processes. Given this and our discussion in section 3 above, it would be reasonable to assert that if our registrars had been general practitioners, we would have found the same lack of statistically significant differences. But tyro and expert clinician are different, and transition from hospital to general practice does present problems for the individual concerned and for the training system. So if differences are not to be found in thinking processes as such, where are they located? In our view, they are to be found in the structure and accessibility of memory, as already illustrated. This conclusion is supported by the empirical work of Neufeld et al (1981) who found in their study that "The only measure of the clinical reasoning process which was consistently related to education level was . . . a measure of the content of the diagnostic hypothesis . . . Furthermore, this measure was the best predictor of the diagnostic outcome. These outcomes were, in turn, strongly correlated with increasing education".

We can see, then, that differences in "expertise" are largely differences in the content, not process, of thinking. However, this does not mean that the "expert" knows more, necessarily. It might just mean that he/she knows differently. That is to say that knowledge and experience might be stored and structured differently in the expert's memory and become more accessible and immediately useable. Forceful features might become more appropriate to the clinical realities of practice and the ways in which patients present. In general practice, memory structures may begin to have greater "management" components or become organised under different "headings" which are broader or less precise than those of the specialist, as with the example given by Brooke et al (1983) of "splitting patients into large binary groups such as urgent/not urgent or upper respiratory infection/lower respiratory infection rather than an exact histological diagnosis". "The Future General Practitioner" (RCGP, 1972) gives another example of the process of restructuring or reorganising knowledge in memory so that it becomes appropriate to clinical practice:

> "(The trainee) will be quick to recognise a raised jugular venous pressure, but slow to interpret a glance of panic which the patient may throw to the doctor in the course of casually mentioning a "minor" symptom. This is partly because "one sees what one knows", and partly because, prior to his entry into the general practice curriculum, the trainee will have accorded higher value to the symptoms and

signs of the physical systems than to those which belong to the psychological and social systems of his patient's life. Now, a proper balance must be learned".

In other words, using the same processes of diagnostic thinking new forceful features must be identified within modified memory structures. We must now turn, finally, to consider psychological explanations of how such changes and modifications occur. Changes in memory structure occur by the complementary mechanisms of assimilation and accommodation as described by Piaget (1952). Assimilation occurs when new information is incorporated into existing memory structures. Example 11 illustrates this.

EXAMPLE 11

Before a ward round, a student's memory structure, concerning steroid therapy side effects might be :

PRE-WARD ROUND MEMORY STRUCTURE

Weight gain
Hypertension
Diabetes
Moon face
"Lemon on toothpicks

On the ward-round, the student sees a patient who has received long term steroids for asthma. The dose has recently been elevated and the patient has become euphoric. Ecchymoses are present in both antecubital fossae. On the basis of this, two new items of information are assimilated into the pre-ward round memory structure.

ASSIMILATION PROCESS

+
Mental change
Easy bruising

ADDITIONAL KNOWLEDGE

Accommodation occurs when the memory structures themselves have to change in order to take account of events in the world. Example 12 illustrates this.

Such processes of assimilation and accommodation will occur inevitably as a result of both formal learning and clinical practice which demands the use of existing memory structures in new conditions.

Although such changes will inevitably occur, we cannot conclude that training programmes are unnecessary! Quite the reverse. The role of training programmes must be central in ensuring that structural changes are achieved efficiently, effectively and appropriately. Complementarily, training programmes should continue to address themselves to the diagnostic thinking processes and psychological factors (see Table 2) which make use of the memory structures. Our identification of 14 thinking processes, associated

EXAMPLE 12
Shown below are two imaginary memory structures which might have been used by a person when he was a medical student and, later, when he practised as a general practitioner in the assessment of the severity of uncontrolled diabetes mellitus in a 50 year old woman who takes gliclazide.

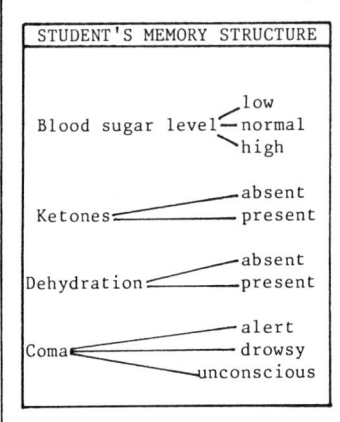

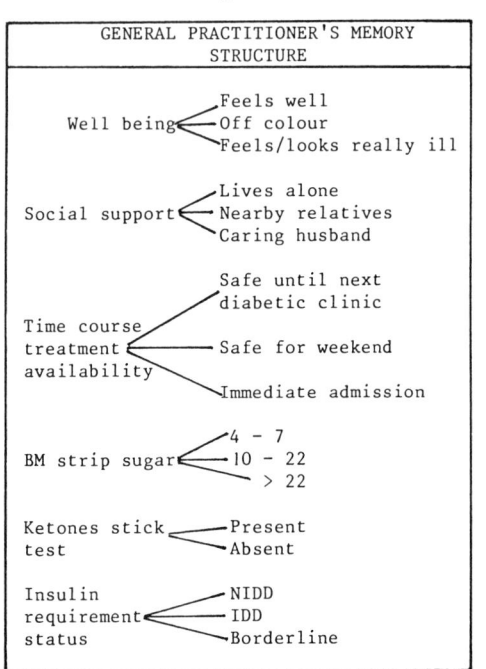

STUDENT'S MEMORY STRUCTURE	GENERAL PRACTITIONER'S MEMORY STRUCTURE
Blood sugar level — low / normal / high	Well being — Feels well / Off colour / Feels/looks really ill
Ketones — absent / present	Social support — Lives alone / Nearby relatives / Caring husband
Dehydration — absent / present	Time course treatment availability — Safe until next diabetic clinic / Safe for weekend / Immediate admission
Coma — alert / drowsy / unconscious	BM strip sugar — 4 - 7 / 10 - 22 / > 22
	Ketones stick test — Present / Absent
	Insulin requirement status — NIDD / IDD / Borderline

We can see here a qualitative change in the way in which information became organised in this clinician's memory. This accommodatory change reflects the different training and experience, needs and practice of the developing clinician. The student's "hospital medicine" structure accommodates to the "general practice" orientated structure. In each, different things are important, different criteria apply. Ketones and blood sugar assume different roles and predominance, for example. Some features disappear, new features appear and the whole structure accommodates.

psychological factors and changing memory structures has led us to conclude that no ideal combination or order of these can be prescribed. The appropriate diagnostic thinking process and content will be dependent upon the circumstance and the individual. We have concluded, therefore, that training programmes can do no other than provide for the learner both structured and unstructured experience of clinical problems, patients, presentations, situations and so on and by analysis and demonstration use these to assist the learner to achieve self-understanding, self-awareness and self-monitoring of his/her own diagnostic thinking processes. In addition, the memory structures and forceful features which the trainee uses can be identified and revealed. We have developed a series of exercises and activities designed to reveal to undergraduate students the items shown in Table 2 as they occur in their own thinking. Such exercises also facilitate analysis of memory structures and planned, appropriate change if necessary. Such a pedagogical approach would be equally as appropriate in general practice training.

REFERENCES

Barrows, H.S., and Bennett, K. (1972) The diagnostic (problem-solving) skill of the neurologist. Archives of Neurology 26, 273-277

Barrows, H.S., Norman, G.R., Neufeld, V.R. and Feightner, J.W. (1978) The clinical reasoning process of the physician. Unpublished report. McMaster University.

Barrows, H.S. and Tamblyn, R.M. (1980) Problem-based learning in medical education. Springer Publishing Co., New York.

Barrows, H.S., Norman, G.R., Neufeld, V.R. and Feightner, J.W. (1982) The clinical reasoning of randomly selected physicians in general medical practice. Clinical and Investigative Medicine, 5, 1, 49-55.

Bentsen, B.G. (1980). The diagnostic process in primary medical care. Primary Care, J. Fry (Ed) Heinemann, London.

Bentsen, B.G. (1984). The health problem and tools for the computer. This publication.

Brooke, J.B., Rector, A.L. and Sheldon, M.G. (1984). A review of studies of decision-making in general practice. Medical Informatics, 9, 45-53.

Brooke, J.B. and Sheldon, M.G. (1985). Decision = patient with problem + doctor with problem. A consideration of general practice decision-making. This publication.

Crombie, D.L. (1963) Diagnostic process. Journal of the College of General Practitioners. 6, 579-589.

Cutler, P. (1979) Problem-Solving in Clinical Medicine. From data to diagnosis. Williams and Wilkins, Baltimore.

Dudley, H.A.F. (1969). Tasks for clinicians : the diagnostic process. Medical Journal of Australia. 1, 37-43

Dudley, H.A.F. (1970) The clinical task. Lancet 2, 1352-1354

Dudley, H.A.F. (1982) Axioms in clinical practice and their potential usefulness in education. Medical Education 16, 308-313

Elstein, A.S. (1976). Clinical judgement : psychological research and medical practice. Science 194, 696-700

Elstein, A.S., Shulman, L.S. and Sprafka, S.A. (1978) Medical Problem Solving : an analysis of clinical reasoning. Harvard University Press, Cambridge, Mass.

Feinstein, A.R. (1967) Clinical judgment. Baltimore : Williams and Wilkins.

Gale, J. (1980) The diagnostic thinking process in medical education and clinical practice. A comparative study of students, house officers and registrars with special reference to endocrinology and neurology. PhD thesis, London University Institute of Education.

Gale, J. (1982) Some cognitive components of the diagnostic thinking process. British Journal of Educational Psychology 52, 64-76.

Gale, J., and Marsden, P. (1982) Clinical problem-solving; the beginning of the process. Medical Education 16, 22-26

Gale, J., and Marsden, P. (1983) Medical Diagnosis : from student to clinician. Oxford University Press, Oxford.

Gorry, G.A. (1970) Modelling the diagnostic process. Journal of Medical Education 45, 292-302

Habbema, J.D.F., and Van der Maas, P.J. (1981). Decision theory in clinical medicine: an appraisal of its uses, its assumptions and its limits. In: Girelli-Bruni, E.(ed) Social, Ideological and Methodological aspects of Medical Statistics. Bertani Editore, Verona, Italy.

Hamilton, M. (1966) Clinicians and Decisions. Leeds University Press

Howie, J.G.R. (1972) Diagnosis - the achilles heel? Journal of the Royal College of General Practitioners 22, 310-315

Howie, J.G.R. (1985) The consultation : a multi-purpose framework. This publication.

Inhelder, B. and Piaget, J. (1958) The growth of logical thinking from childhood to adolescence. London: Routledge and Kegan Paul.

Keighley, M.R.B., Hoare, A.M., Horrocks, J.C., De Dombal, F.T. and Alexander, W.J. (1976) A symptomatic discriminant to identify recurrent ulcer patients with dyspepsia after gastric surgery. Lancet 2, 278-279.

Kleinmuntz, B. (1968) Formal representation of human judgement. New York: Wiley.

Knafl, K. and Burkett, G. (1975) Professional socialisation in a surgical specialty: acquiring medical judgement. Social Science and Medicine 9, 397-404.

Knill-Jones, R.P. (1975) The diagnosis of jaundice by the computation of probabilities. Journal of the Royal College of Physicians of London 205-210

Knill-Jones, R.P. (1977) Clinical decision-making (2) Diagnostic and prognostic inference. Health Bulletin 35, July/September, 213-222.

Mayou, R. (1978) Psychiatric decision-making by medical students. British Journal of Psychiatry 132, 191-194

Meals, R.A. (1973) Teaching clinical judgement. British Journal of Medical Education 7, 100-102

Medawar, P.B. (1969) Induction and Intuition in Scientific Thought. London: Methuen & Co.Ltd.

McWhinney, I.R. (1972) Problem-solving and decision-making in primary medical practice. Proceedings of the Royal Society of Medicine 65, 934-938.

McWhinney, I.R. (1980) Decision-making in general practice. Journal of the Royal College of General Practitioners. Occasional paper 10.

Murray, T.S., Cupples, R.W., Barber, J.H., Dunn, W.R., Scott, D.B. and Hannay, D.R. (1977) Teaching decision-making to medical undergraduates by computer-assisted learning. Medical Education 11, 262-264.

Neufeld, V.R., Norman, G.R., Feightner, J.W. and Barrows, H.S. (1981) Clinical problem-solving by medical students : a cross-sectional and longitudinal analysis. Medical Education 15, 315-322

Neutra, R. (1977) Indications for the surgical treatment of suspected acute appendicitis: A cost-effectiveness approach, 277-307. In: Costs, Risks and Benefits of Surgery. Bunker, J.P., Barnes, B.A. and Mosteller, F. (eds) Oxford University Press, New York.

Pauker, S.G., Gorry, G.A., Kassirer, J.P. and Schwarz, W.B. (1976) Towards the simulation of clinical cognition. Taking a present illness by computer. American Journal of Medicine 60, 981-996

Piaget, J. (1952) The origins of intelligence in children. New York : International University Press.

Ridderikhoff, J. (1982) Research into decision-making strategies used in general practice. Proceedings of Medical Informatics Europe '82, 16, 272-279.

Ridderikhoff, J. (1985) The paper patient. A device for investigation in general practice. This publication.

Royal College of General Practitioners (1972) The Future General Practitioner. Learning and Teaching. Published for the R.C.G.P. by the British Medical Journal, London.

Scadding, J.G. (1967) Diagnosis : the clinician and the computer. The Lancet 1, 877-882.

Schwarz, W.B., Gorry, G.A., Kassirer, J.P. and Essig, A. (1973) Decision analysis and clinical judgement. American Journal of Medicine 55, 459-472.

Sprafka, S.A. and Elstein, A.S. (1974) What do physicians do? An analysis of diagnostic reasoning. Paper presented at the OMERAD symposium on medical judgement. Michigan State University, East Lansing.

Style, A. (1979) Intuition and problem-solving. Journal of the Royal College of General Practitioners 29, 71-74.

Taylor, T.R., Aitchison, J. and McGirr, E.M. (1971) Doctors as decision-makers. A computer-assisted study of diagnosis as a cognitive skill. British Medical Journal 3, 35-40.

8
Discussion of the Paper by Gale and Marsden

Frank Martin Hull

The discussion following this paper on "Diagnosis: Process not Product" was influenced by the nature of the group and the position it had reached as a result of the reading and presentations up to this point in the conference.

The heterogeneity of the group, drawn from many disciplines, each with a spectrum from the pragmatist to the theorist, ensured that each of us saw the problem of decision-making from a different viewpoint. It was as though there were a piece of truth at the centre of us but because each of us had a different viewpoint, so seeing that truth from a different angle, we could not recognise it for what it was. This lack of recognition was compounded by the swirling mists of different preconceptions, semantics and thought processes within each observer.

A further problem, already referred to by Howie and created by the heterogeneity of the group was that each delegate sought something different from the conference. Some practising doctors, anxious to improve their own proficiency at decision-making, took a clinical stance. Others, seeking a better preparation for new generations of entrants to general practice, asked how they could become better teachers. Still others, the thinkers and theorists, sought a simple formula, a theoretical framework encapsulating the principle of decision-making in order, in McWhinney's words, to tie facts into neat bundles for classification and ease of teaching. A fourth group, from the world of the computer, sought to explain decision-making in terms compatible with their technology.

These then, appeared to be the viewpoints and objectives of the groups to whom Doctors Gale and Marsden gave their fascinating paper with such excellent and skilfully stage managed delivery. In this discussion five aspects could be discerned: clarification of terms, followed by the views of clinicians, teachers, theorists and those familiar with computer technology.

Clarification of Terms

The terms giving rise to most difficulty were 'content', 'pattern recognition' and 'forceful feature'. 'Content' referred to the doctor's thought which in turn was dependent on his memory bank with which he interpreted data as he gathered it, constantly re-interpreting it in the light of new information.

There was difficulty in distinguishing between 'pattern recognition' and the 'forceful feature'. The former has, in the past, been badly and loosely used. The authors explained it as a sudden event implying active involvement by the physician as a result of one or more forceful features which stimulated active thought so leading to a congruence of stored or observed data and its organisation and recognition as a familiar pattern. The 'forceful feature' is an intrapsychic event, a subjective identification of a special item of information in conjunction with data in memory which, alone or with others, may initiate pattern recognition.

Views of Clinicians

Pragmatic general practitioners welcomed this concept with cases from their own experience. The need for decision very early in the consultation is characteristic of primary care and depends on the simultaneous appreciation of information derived from the doctors knowledge of the environment (the background) against which the patient's presenting symptom and the doctor's previous knowledge of the patient are weighed. As a result of this the doctor decides the seriousness of the problem and how much diagnostic effort he will spend upon it. An example was given of a general practitioners observation of a dairy farmer's herd being reduced in number and the ploughing of good pasture. These were not forceful features, but were noticed by a curious doctor and stored in his memory. When later the dairyman presented in mid-summer with 'flu' this was a forceful feature and stimulated the recognition of the pattern of acute brucellosis.

The Views of Teachers

Teachers expressed some concern about the concept, wondering how it would help them to teach students to make speedy, accurate decisions. It was suggested that the thrust of the paper, particularly with its reference to research on hospital based clinicians, was directed towards traditional, doctor-centred medicine. The difference between general practice and hospital medicine had previously led to discussion in which it was felt that there was a difference but that far too much stress had been put upon this since both forms of medicine lay within the continuum of a spectrum. It was suggested that there was imbalance of emphasis in the paper for it was neither product nor process that were important so much as the problem from which the process stemmed. Teachers were also interested in the practical application: how was the theory used in teaching and how was it received by the taught? This was the subject of further study by the authors, but their early experience showed that, after initial difficulty students accepted the idea thoughtfully, found that they analysed their thinking processes and came to like the teaching.

The View of the Theoreticians

It was asked whether this was a theory of clinical knowledge rather than thinking (denied by the authors) and whether the theory applied generally to, say, stockbrokers - if it were general could it actually be taught or did one need brain damage to undergo so radical a change? The authors suspected that there was a commonality of thinking between different kinds of people but this was another area of intended research. It was asked whether the theory had power to predict thinking processes, but Gale and Marsden explained that the description was not proscriptive since individuals would select those particular subsets of thinking processes as they personally needed during any one consultation; this is largely unpredictable. All that is known is that individuals have a range of thinking processes available to them.

The theory was summed up epigrammatically as: we can't think much about our learning, but we can learn a lot about our thinking.

The Technological View

Some criticism was implied at deficiency of the extensive artificial intelligence amd computer based literature in the paper, but such deficiency was the result of selection rather than omission. This had arisen because of the authors' distinction between the process and content of thought which was not acceptable to the technologist who admitted that he was thinking computing terms. The authors insisted that memory was accessed through forceful features which had nothing to do with the objective identification or predetermined arrangement, or adding of content: this remained unsatisfactory to the computer expert.

Finally there was a warning from a general practitioner that over analysis of an acquired intuitive skill could lead to a tidy theory and coincidentally destroy the previously unexplained ability. Caution was urged, lest we damaged the very thing we sought to understand and preserve.

9
Clinical Decision = Patient with Problem + Doctor with Problem

J.B. Brooke and M.G. Sheldon

INTRODUCTION

Decision-making in general practice is not a simple matter of a patient presenting a problem and the doctor making a rational, correct decision. The human skills of decision-making are often poor, although at the moment still better than automated decision-making, especially where the problem is ill-defined.

There is little reason to think that doctors are any more skilled at making decisions within their own area of expertise than are businessmen about financial matters or car mechanics about the origin of funny noises under the bonnet. Decision-making itself is a problem and making correct decisions is a skill that must be learnt. Teaching that skill, in turn, requires an understanding of the underlying process.

In recent years much research has been directed towards the study of medical decision-making. Reviews of the literature in the area (eg. Elstein et al., 1978; Taylor, 1980) indicate that the emphasis of this research has been on decision-making in hospital settings. Relatively few studies consider the ways in which decisions are made in general practice.

Several authors have pointed out that there are important differences between general practice and hospital practice (Howie, 1972; McWhinney, 1972; Bentsen, 1980). It is not the intention of this paper to explore these differences in detail; a composite list of differences has been given elsewhere (Brooke, Rector and Sheldon, 1984). However, some of the salient differences are

- a general practitioner sees a much wider range of problems;
- problems are presented in an undifferentiated fashion;

- psychosocial problems play a far greater role in general practice;

- the probabilities and presentation of diseases are different;

- the general practitioner has a much more personal and continuing relationship with his patient;

- there are shorter, more frequent contacts rather than fewer, longer contacts as in the hospital setting.

CURRENT MODELS OF GENERAL PRACTICE DECISION-MAKING

Models or frameworks of general practice decision-making do exist (McWhinney, 1972, 1980; Ridderikhof, 1982). These models are largely of a sequential nature; that is, they assume that decision-making consists of a number of stages, and that the doctor proceeds from one stage to another in an orderly fashion, possibly returning to earlier stages to revise a decision but then following the main sequence again. The models bear close resemblance to other models of decision-making such as those of Elstein et al., (1972, 1978).

These models tend to concentrate on the diagnostic decision-making task. Diagnosis in general practice is a rather fuzzy concept and does not necessarily need to be of a high level of precision in order to select the appropriate management (Crombie, 1963; Hull, 1969, 1972). In fact much of the emphasis in general practice is on management rather than on diagnosis. Howie (1972) suggests that the quality of care delivered in general practice might be improved if doctors did not attempt to give their patients the sort of diagnostic tag they have been trained to use by their hospital specialist teachers.

It is perhaps surprising that these models do not emphasise the role of management. It has been pointed out that one of the distinguishing features of general practice is that management is a major component of the diagnostic cycle (Bentsen, 1980). General practitioners use both deferral of decision (a passive form of management) and trials of therapy as diagnostic tools. In this sense, diagnosis as an end product of the consultation may often be completely irrelevant, since by the time a diagnosis is reached using these strategies, the management will either have been effective or the patient will be recovering anyway despite the management. On this basis, there is no way of ever knowing whether the diagnosis was in fact correct; and anyway it often doesn't matter very much. It is management that matters.

The models of general practice decision-making are however distinctive for their explanations of how general practitioners cope with the wide range of problems that confront them. One strategy that has been suggested is that of early problem closure (McWhinney, 1972, 1980). This suggests that rather than considering the total range of diagnoses that might apply to a patient, the doctor quickly hypothesises a limited number of possible diagnoses and then proceeds to test these hypotheses only. This contrasts with the strategy of progressive reduction of the complete range of diagnoses that Kleinmuntz (1968) puts forward as a model of expert decision-making.

Ridderikhof (1982) proposes that the formation of hypotheses takes place as pattern recognition, and that pattern recognition is often the only step necessary in making a decision. However, with more complex problems, the doctor may switch to a sequential 'deductive' strategy.

Both the strategy of problem closure and the use of inductive pattern directed search and heuristics are causes for concern. Elstein and co workers (1972) talk of the 'dangers inherent in early hypothesis generation' and suggest that traditional routinised medical practices such as history-taking and examination safeguard against consideration of completely incorrect hypotheses. The confidence one has in decisions made on this basis depends on one's perceptions of the quality of the human as decision-maker.

SHORTCOMINGS OF HUMANS AS DECISION-MAKERS

There is a good deal of evidence that humans are not necessarily very good decision-makers, and that in limited areas they can be outperformed by fairly simple automated decision-making systems (de Dombal, 1972; Cohen, 1979). Research on decision-making in a number of areas other than medicine has identified a dizzying collection of sources of cognitive bias. Sage (1981), in a comprehensive review of the literature on decision-making research, lists no less than twenty-seven sources of cognitive bias which can lead to a decrement in the quality of decision-making. There is no reason to think that this list is exhaustive. It includes such things as the tendency of decision-makers to use only easily available information and to ignore that which is less accessible; a failure to satisfactorily revise estimates of probability when presented with new information due to conservatism; the use of heuristics to cope with information overload; and the influence of order of presentation of information on its retention in memory, which in turn affects the way in which decisions are made.

As Sage points out, these results are disturbing in that they ". . . imply that humans may be little more than masters of the art of self-deception" (1981, p.649). Although these results have been obtained from the study of decision-making largely outside the medical context, there is no reason to suppose that medical practitioners do not suffer from the same types of bias.

Another shortcoming of present models of decision-making is their generality. Taylor (1980), discussing sequential models of medical decision-making, points out that they are unlikely to be a complete model of all the intellectual processes involved in clinical decisions. He suggests that 'it is more likely to represent the most easily accessible cognitive functions of the clinician'. However, he suggests that in both clinical and business decision-making, it is far more common to find an apparent pattern recognition solution to problems. Post hoc rationalisations of these intuitive decisions may be made in terms of a sequential model at a later stage.

PROBLEMS, PROBLEM-SOLVERS, AND PROBLEM-SOLVING STRATEGIES

A second source of concern arising from these models of general practice decision-making is that they assume a consistent mechanism which applies across a range of problems. However, there is a need to consider the role played by the problem presented in determining the method of its own solution. Elstein (1978), studying clinical decision-making under laboratory conditions, failed to distinguish between 'good' and 'bad' diagnosticians. Rather, there was considerable variation in the quality of problem solution within individual doctors, and a far larger proportion of the variance in the problem-solving strategies was attributable to the nature of the problems set rather than to variations between doctors' problem-solving styles.

Sage's review of decision-making research (1981) considers the topic of 'cognitive style' in some depth and comes to a similar conclusion; that is, the characteristics of the decision-making task seem to be the prime determinant of decision-making strategy.

Some workers have found that, given similar medical problems, different specialists (Bloor, 1978) and different general practitioners (Raynes, 1980) develop different strategies for coping. This would seem to indicate some interaction between the nature of the problem and the problem-solving style of the doctor. However, it may equally well indicate different interpretations of the same problem; one doctor may see a problem as being purely organic, while another sees the same problem as being psychosocial. These differing interpretations may lead to different solution strategies.

In view of the fact that one of the distinguishing features of general practice is the wide range of problems encompassed, it is critical for the study of decision-making that we gain insight into the nature of the different problems encountered and the ways in which they modify the decision-making task.

WHAT CONSTITUTES A DECISION PROBLEM IN GENERAL PRACTICE?

There are a number of approaches to this question. In a recent study in this department we tried to identify decision problems by identifying those clinical areas in which general practitioners express some uncertainty about aspects of their judgement during the consultation. A group of forty-two general practitioners made ratings on a five point scale of their certainty about diagnosis, the completeness of the history they had taken, and the appropriateness of the management they had selected in one hundred consecutive surgery consultations. The use of the three certainty rating scales is shown in Figure 1.

FIG. 1
CERTAINTY RATING SCALES

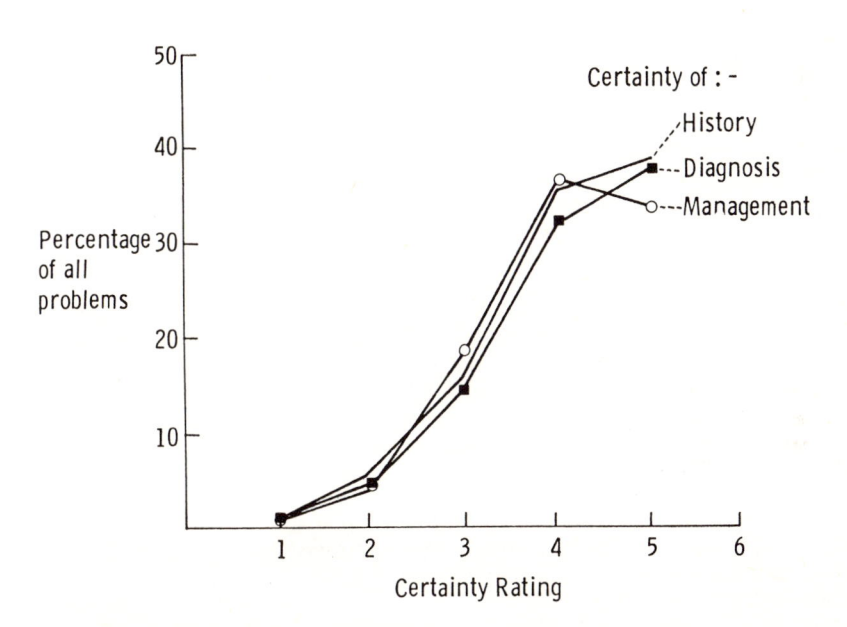

[Graph showing percentage of all problems (y-axis, 0-50) versus Certainty Rating (x-axis, 1-6) for three curves: History, Diagnosis, and Management]

On all three rating scales, the fourth and fifth point was used in 70-75% of all cases. The fifth point (ie. 'very certain') was used most commonly on the history and diagnosis certainty scales and the fourth point on the management certainty scale.

In general, a certainty rating of three or less was used in about 25% of all cases on all of the scales. We have therefore adopted the convention that a rating of three or less on a scale indicates some degree of uncertainty about that aspect of the case.

Three clinical areas led to a high rate of uncertainty in all three aspects of problem solution. These were gastrointestinal problems, neurological problems and musculoskeletal problems, especially those of a spinal or rheumatic nature.

Certain clinical areas led to high rates on some, but not all, aspects of the case. Gynaecological problems (excluding those to do with contraception or pregnancy) commonly led to uncertainty about management. Another area of high uncertainty was the diagnosis and management of upper respiratory tract problems. This last area of uncertainty suggests that when uncertainty is expressed it does not necessarily mean that the doctor has a problem. The doctor may think that the patient with a runny nose and slightly elevated temperature is suffering from a virus infection. He may not be sure about this, and he may be even less certain as to which virus is responsible. However, it will not lead to a decision-making problem because even if no action is taken then the balance of probabilities is for a good prognosis.

Gastrointestinal problems, on the other hand, constitute an important area of uncertainty in general practice decision-making. The risks to the patient consequent to an incorrect diagnosis or course of management are high. Equally, over-reaction in management by referring too early can be excessively costly. This has long been recognised as an area of deficiency in decision-making, and it has become one in which attention has been concentrated on providing decision support systems (Knill-Jones and Dunwoodie, 1985; de Dombal, 1972).

Musculoskeletal problems can be awkward for other reasons. Often the decision the doctor faces is to do with the management of chronic pain from causes such as arthritis, or pain of an ill-defined nature, as with low back pain. There is relatively little uncertainty about the diagnosis of rheumatic complaints, probably reflecting their chronic nature; but there is high uncertainty about their management. The sources of uncertainty about management are not clear, but one might speculate that because these problems are typically diseases of late middle aged and elderly patients, there may be other problems which interact with the management of the rheumatic problem. Thus use of a simple anti-inflammatory such as aspirin may be ruled out because of co-existing gastrointestinal conditions. In fact, as we shall see in the section below, general practitioners commonly consider musculoskeletal presentations to be decision-making problems in their own right, but less commonly when seen in conjunction with other physiological problems.

It is obvious that there are a number of underlying causes of uncertainty in general practice problems which need to be clarified. A second approach we have used to study the range and nature of decison-making problems is to ask general practitioners what they themselves consider to be the salient features of these problems.

GENERAL PRACTITIONERS' PERCEPTIONS OF DECISION-MAKING PROBLEMS

We have undertaken a study of general practitioners' perceptions of clinical decisions which employed the repertory grid technique. This technique provides qualitative information about the structure of an individual's perceptions of the world about him. For a full description of the technique the interested reader is referred to the work of Fransella and Bannister (1977). Essentially, each of the twelve doctors participating in this study collected a sample of cases they felt were 'interesting decision-making problems' and were then interviewed using a highly structured technique, in which they were asked what they felt were important points of difference between the cases.

The types of case selected as being 'interesting from a decision-making point of view corresponded quite closely to those identified in the study of uncertainty previously discussed. Once again, gynaecological, musculoskeletal and gastrointestinal problems were the most commonly selected. However, there were some interesting differences in terms of whether problems occurred singly or in combinations. Gynaecological and musculoskeletal problems tended to appear singly and thus appear to constitute decision-making problems in their own right. Gastrointestinal problems, on the other hand, were very commonly selected when occurring with other physiological problems or with psychosocial problems. Cardiovascular problems were also commonly selected but these were more commonly associated with psychosocial problems in the cases presented in this study.

There thus seems to be a fairly consistent picture of areas of uncertainty in general practice decision-making which have been identified by both direct and indirect means. In particular, musculoskeletal, gynaecological and gastrointestinal problems are the main areas of concern.

When doctors were interviewed about their perceptions of the important distinguishing features of these problems, a certain polarity emerged between those who concentrated on the human aspects of the problem and those who were concerned with the problems per se. A doctor on the human-oriented side of this continuum might say that an important feature of some problems was that there were people other than the patient who might be affected by the outcome of the decision. A doctor who was "problem-oriented" might say that the most important feature of some decision-making problems was that decisions had to be made about the choice between several competing types of drug therapy.

This 'human-centred' versus 'problem-centred' distinction is one that fits quite well with anecdotal evidence. Whilst the majority of general practitioners studied fell somewhere between the two poles, there were some 'extreme' cases. A matter of interest for research is the extent to which the doctors' decision-making strategies are affected by their position on the continuum, and how it relates to the type of problem presented to them.

One of the most common distinctions made between decision-making problems was that in some the problem is ill-defined whilst in others it is well-defined. Correlates of poor problem definition included multiple problems being presented simultaneously; psychological problems more commonly being seen as being ill-defined; and for several doctors there was a correlation between poor problem definition and a bad doctor-patient relationship. It is difficult to tease out any sort of cause and effect from the qualitative data of this study. There are equally good explanations that the doctor grows to dislike patients who persistently present vague problems or that because the doctor dislikes the patient, the patient cannot communicate the nature of his problem adequately. The work reported by Hull (1985) would tend to indicate that patients feel that doctors do not understand their problems anyway. This situation may be made worse if the patient perceives that their doctor dislikes them.

Another common distinction that doctors drew between decision-making problems was based on the clinical areas into which the problems fell. Thus, decisions about orthopaedic problems were seen as being different to decisions about non-orthopaedic problems by some doctors. Others perceived important differences between cases which involved menstrual problems and those which did not. These distinctions were frequently correlated with other dimensions of difference such as 'some problems are largely about diagnosis; others are largely to do with management'. However, the correlates of particular clinical distinctions varied from doctor to doctor. An interesting question for future research would be to investigate whether there is any consensus about the distinguishing features of decisions in particular problem areas. Are menstrual problems distinguished by problems of diagnosis? Is the management of pain one of the things that makes orthopaedic problems difficult?

The last distinction commonly made that we will deal with here was that between some problems being of an organic nature whilst others were of a psychological nature. As pointed out above, the prominence of psychosocial problems is commonly held to be one of the distinguishing features of general practice. What effect does this aspect of the nature of problems have on the way in which decisions are made? As we have seen in the discussion of problem definition, the presence of psychological problems is a correlate of what some doctors consider to be poorly defined problems. There must, however, be other distinguishing features of psychosocial problems.

WHY DO WE NEED MODELS OF DECISION-MAKING?

These studies raise a number of questions about general practice decision-making. More important are the questions they raise about why we want to create models of the decision-making process and what the nature of these models should be.

It would appear that there is no one approach to decision-making, and there are many other degrees of freedom involved in determination of the decision-making process. Can we, and indeed should we attempt to unify all these different appraoches into a single model? This question is answerable only if we consider the reasons for producing a model of decision-making. One reason might be that we are dissatisfied with the quality of decisions that are currently being made and we may wish to improve them, either by education of the decision-maker, or by intervening and passing part or all of the decision to a decision support system. Alternatively, we may think that some practitioners are good decision-makers and that we wish to persuade others to emulate their approach to decision-making. If the latter case applies, then we have a case for producing a single model of decision-making. It will only reflect one possible approach to the problem, but we will have selected it because we have somehow judged it to be a 'good' approach.

If, on the other hand, we think that decisions could actually be made rather better than they are at present, and that there are no experts, then the case for a single model is rather weaker. What we should perhaps be looking for is an admission that different problems need different solutions, and that different doctors deal with them in different ways. Rather than a model of decision-making, we should have a collection of all the strategies, all the search schemes, all the management plans and all the mechanisms for coping with interpersonal problems; then we should try and provide some mechanism by which we can recognise shortcomings in decision-making strategies and select alternative approaches. For this reason, the work of Essex (1985) is of great interest as he is attempting to provide this appraoch in general practice education.

CONCLUSIONS

The topic of decision-making in general practice is even more complicated than it might at first appear. For a number of reasons, simple sequential decision models seem inappropriate for the types of problem that are faced, not the least of which is that different problems require very different strategies for solution; and the range of problems in general practice is enormous. There is also evidence of distinct differences in the ways in which general practitioners approach problems, and this can interact with the range of problems to give an even wider range of models that could be adopted.

The variance in problem-solving strategies, and the feeling that humans are not, in any case, optimal decision-makers leads the authors to conclude that perhaps general models of decision-making in this field are not desirable. Research could instead be concentrated on collecting different approaches to problems and on the description of rules and heuristics for selecting the most appropriate approach to each particular set of problems.

REFERENCES

Bentsen, B. G., (1980) 'The Diagnostic Process in Primary Medical Care,' in Primary Care, J. Fry (Ed.), London, Heinemann.

Bloor, M., (1978) 'On the Routinised Nature of Work in People Processing Agencies,' in Relationships between Doctors and Patients, Davis (Ed.), London, Saxon House.

Brooke, J. B., Rector, A. L. and Sheldon, M. G. (1984), 'A Review of Studies of Decision-Making in General Practice,' Medical Informatics, 9, 45-53.

Cohen, L. J. (1979), 'On the Psychology of Prediction: Whose is the Fallacy,' Cognition, 7, 385-407.

Crombie, D. L. (1963), 'Diagnostic Process,' Journal of the Royal College of General Practitioners, 6, 579-589.

de Dombal, F. T. (1972), 'Computers and the Surgeon - A Matter of Decision,' Surgery Annual, 11, 33-57.

Elstein, A. S., Kagan, N., Shulman, L. S., Jason, H. and Loupe, M. (1972), 'Methods and Theory in the Study of Medical Enquiry,' J. Medical Education, 47, 85-97.

Elstein, A. S. Shulman, L. S. and Sprafka, S. A. (1978), Medical Problem-Solving, Cambridge, Mass., Harvard Press.

Essex, B. (1985)   This volume.

Fransella, F. and Bannister, D. (1977), A Manual for Repertory Grid Technique, London, Academic Press.

Howie, J. G. R. (1972), 'Diagnosis - The Achilles Heel?' Journal of the Royal College of General Practitioners.

Hull, F. M. (1969), 'Diagnostic Pathways in Rural General Practice, Journal of the Royal College of General Practitioners, 18, 148-155.

Hull, F. M. (1972), 'Diagnostic Pathways in General Practice,' Journal of the Royal College of General Practitioners, 22, 241-258.

Hull, F.M. (1985)   This volume.

Kleinmuntz, B. (1968), 'The Processing of Clinical Information by Man and Machine.'   In: Formal Representation of Human Judgement, B. Kleinmuntz (Ed.), New York, John Wiley.

Knill-Jones, R. P., and Dunwoodie, W. M. (1985)   This volume.

McWhinney, I. R. (1972), 'Problem-Solving and Decision-Making in Primary Medical Practice,' Proceedings Royal Society of Medicine, 65, 934-938.

McWhinney, I. R. (1980), 'Decision-Making in General Practice,' Journal of the Royal College of General Practitioners, Occasional Paper 10. 31-33.

Raynes, N. V. (1980), 'A Preliminary Study of Search Procedures and Patient Management in General Practice,' Journal of the Royal College of General Practitioners, 30, 166-172.

Ridderikhoff, J. (1982), 'Research into Decision-making Strategies used General Practice,' Proceedings of Medical Informatics Europe 82, 16, 272-279.

Sage, A. P. (1981) 'Behavioural and Organisational Considerations in the Design of Information Systems and Processes for Planning and Decision Support,' IEEE Transaction on Systems, Man and Cybernetics, SMC-11, 640-678.

Taylor, T. (1980), 'The Role of Computer Systems in Medical Decision-making,' in Human Interaction with Computers, H. Smith and T. R. G. Green (Eds.), London, Academic Press.

10
Knowledge and Judgement in Decision-making

John Fox

INTRODUCTION

Although faced with a wide range of medical problems, and working under conditions of limited resources and constant technical change, the GP is expected to manage patients quickly and well. This contradiction attracts a variety of proposed solutions. Some people look for more resources, some emphasise better training and others better organisation. This paper considers whether computer technology can be used to amplify one of the basic skills of the GP; that of decision-making.

Many types of computer system can help in making decisions. Databases store and recall patient records; statistical techniques can be used to identify practice trends or assess individual risk factors, and so on. However, I am not concerned here with data-processing techniques which simply inform the GP - they can add to rather than reduce the level of work. Decision technology goes beyond data processing - it embodies a theory of what decisions are and methods for taking them. A computer can be used as a tool in deciding what, if anything, is wrong with a patient and what, if any, action to take.

Decision technology must be competent and it must be acceptable. It must be competent to improve the accuracy of diagnosis, the selection of treatments, or help to achieve other clinical goals. Competent decision-making theories based on statistics have been available for about twenty years. Surprisingly, however, the techniques have had little impact (Spiegelhalter and Knill-Jones, 1984). I believe that the techniques may have failed primarily because they are not acceptable; they impose a view of clinical decision-making which is unnatural to the clinician (Fox, 1983).

TOWARDS "NATURAL" DECISION-MAKING

Most decision concepts, and strategies for decision-taking, have their roots in mathematics, notably probability theory. In recent years a new kind of system has emerged which is informal and often non-mathematical. These are "knowledge-based" or "expert" systems. Medical expert systems have been designed which can advise on possible diagnoses, investigation selection and treatment planning (Duda and Shortliffe, 1983; Fox and Alvey, 1983). Figure 1 illustrates a short consultation with a knowledge- based system for advising on the management of terminal patients (under development by P. Alvey and the author).

```
----------PATIENT-1----------
1) Name:
** FRED SMITH
2) What problems are troubling Fred Smith?
** DYSPNOEA
3) What is the severity of the dyspnoea?
** MILD
4) Does Fred Smith have bronchospasm?
** YES
5) Is Fred Smith taking any medication?
** NO
6) Does Fred Smith have a pleural effusion?
** NO
7) Does Fred Smith have anaemia?
** UNK
8) Does Fred Smith have a mediastinal tumour?
** NO
```

Advice for DYSPNOEA
    Steroids are the most effective treatment for bronchospasm (the long term effects are not important in terminal patients).
    Investigate the possibility of anaemia if its correction would improve Fred Smith's personal or family life.

General Advice for DYSPNOEA
    Oxygen is not recommended (because it does not usually ease the dyspnoea of terminal patients).

FIGURE 1

An example of a consultation using the ICRF terminal care system. The user has indicated that the patient is suffering from dyspnoea or breathlessness. (User input follows the ** prompts, all other lines were typed by the system.) The user entered UNK in response to question 7 to indicate that the answer is unknown. A feature of many systems is that only questions relevant to the current problem are asked, so consultations are only as long as is necessary. Other consultations may be longer and more comprehensive.

Why are expert systems different from their predecessors? It is often said that an expert system "mimics" the thought processes of a human expert (at least to a first approximation). For example, there is an emphasis on qualitative reasoning to arrive at a decision, in preference to quantitative techniques. Knowledge is often represented as "rules" and "facts" rather than as mathematical probabilities or utilities. These features help to make expert systems intelligible.

A further attractive feature is that, to a degree, expert systems are able to provide explanations of their actions. If a doctor is unhappy about a recommended decision, or about questions the computer has asked, an explanation of the system's reasoning can be requested, and a judgment made about its validity. Figure 2 illustrates an explanation facility.

Although important the explanation feature and the attempt to mimic human thought are not invariable in expert systems. One feature that must be present for a decision aid to be called an expert system in my view is that the knowledge it uses is explicit; it is not implicit in some abstract model or in the structure of the computer program.

EXPLICIT REPRESENTATION OF MEDICAL KNOWLEDGE

Compare the mathematical approach to representing medical information to the knowledge-based approach. Typically a statistical system for decision-making employs a table of "conditional probabilities", which represents the frequencies with which events co-occur, like the frequency of co-occurrence of diseases and symptoms. These numbers represent a relationship between the symptoms and diseases, but in a very abstract form. They say nothing about what a symptom is, what a disease is, whether "cholecystitis" is a symptom or a disease, or whether a symptom is caused by a disease or just statistically associated with it. Each number records the scale of a relationship but not its sense.

In knowledge engineering, we try to represent knowledge in a way that preserves the natural sense as well as the scale of relationships. One way of doing this is by storing the relationships as explicit "facts" like:

        duodenal-ulcer is-a-kind-of peptic ulcer

        duodenum is-a-part-of gi-system

        ulceration is-a-cause-of bleeding

If the relationship is not clear-cut we may need to quantify it with numbers or in some other way. Here are some examples:

    gastric-cancer is-associated-with weight-loss (.7)

cholecystitis is-associated-with severe-pain (usually)

oesophagitis is-usually-associated-with reflux

The ability to exploit the sense of the relationship as well as its numerical magnitude gives expert systems their potential for

```
7) Does Fred Smith have dyspepsia?
** WHY
```

[i.e. WHY is it important to determine whether PATIENT-1 has dyspepsia?]

[1.0] This will aid in determining whether PATIENT-1 is suspected of having a peptic ulcer.
    If
        [1.1] 1) Fred Smith has dyspepsia, or
            2) Fred Smith has evidence of gastro-intestinal haemorrhage
    then
        it is definite (1.0) that Fred Smith is suspected of having a peptic ulcer
    [RULE020]

```
[back to question 7...]
** WHY
```

[i.e. WHY is it important to determine whether PATIENT-1 is suspected of having a peptic ulcer?]

[2.0]... in order to determine the recommendations for pain.
    It has already been established that
        [2.1] an anti-inflammatory drug should be recommended for Fred Smith, and
        [2.2] oral drugs are suitable for Fred Smith
    Therefore, if
        [2.3] Fred Smith is not suspected of having a peptic ulcer
    then
        it is definite (1.0) that the following is one of the recommendations for pain: Aspirin orally
    [RULE079]

```
[back to question 7...]
** NO
```

FIGURE 2

The explanation facility of EMYCIN, a package designed at Stanford University for developing expert systems. The user was puzzled when asked if his patient has dyspepsia (indigestion), so instead of answering immediately he entered the command WHY. The second WHY produced an explanation at the next higher level in the logical process.

intelligibility. In addition, it is valuable because it is a rich
source of information. For example, knowledge of causal relationships
may let us account for observations or suggest new hypotheses (duodenal
ulcers cause bleeding but not vice versa). "Inheritance" of properties
among members of classes can lead to valuable generalisations (duodenal
and gastric ulcers inherit generic properties of ulcers). Logical
constraints can be used for planning (a drug which may exacerbate one
of the patient's problems is undesirable). Furthermore, many processes
need to be described over time (events can be described as before,
after, during, simultaneous etc.). In many fields, even those as
imprecise as medicine, the qualitative element is usually at least as
important as the quantitative one and needs to be reflected in our
decision-making techniques.

This process of making knowledge explicit does not stop here in the
static or "declarative" part of the knowledge base. In expert systems
it is often extended into the "procedural" parts of the system,
primarily by including rules in the knowledge base. Rules describe
actions within the general format "IF this THEN do that". Another way
of viewing rules is to see them as exploiting the logical relationship
of implication; the conditions are logical premises and when they are
true then the action is to draw a conclusion.

When we define rules we are applying the idea of explication again.
This time we are making the process of reasoning itself explicit, and
the reasoning of the computer becomes more like that of a doctor. It
also yields the potential for accountability - we can see how a
conclusion is arrived at, and judge it critically.

DECISIONS

The expert systems which have been developed for medical
application have shown that the explicit use of knowledge in the form
of rules and facts can give considerable competence in specialised
fields. They also represent an important step towards systems which
are intelligible and accountable to the user by presenting the rules
which are used to make decisions in acceptable English. However,
although the systems may soon be acceptable for use in specialised
clinical settings, the techniques developed so far are probably still
inapplicable when one considers the traditions and practices of the GP
(Fox and Rector, 1982).

Brooke et al. (1984) summarise some of the ways in which GP
decision-making differs from speciality decision-making. Their list
includes the wide range of ill-defined problems, the lower precision
that is needed, the short and frequent pattern of encounters and the
greater range of information the GP has about the patient's background.

At this level of decision-making there is no theory available for
the GP to draw upon, judgment must be used. There is consequently no
theory for the decision technologist to follow either. In this respect

Brooke et al. (1983) offer a suggestive analysis of GP decision-making based upon a study of doctors' own knowledge of their decision-making problems. They show the heterogeneity of decision aspects (diagnosis related, management related, problem related, patient related) and also ways in which these aspects may interact in the doctor's mind. In short, it is not sufficient to view medical decision-making simply as using objective rules and facts to interpret data. We need to have a clearer idea of what we mean by decisions and, most importantly, judgments.

Consider the problem of the patient who repeatedly visits his doctor complaining of vague dyspepsia, but who is known to have distressing family problems. The GP may view his task not of defining an exact diagnosis but of deciding whether to recommend antacids or counselling, whether to temporise or refer the patient. There are at least two levels of decision-making here, the classic one of deciding the diagnosis (when appropriate) and also a higher level judgment - that of deciding whether to attempt a diagnosis at all or to take some other action, such as arranging a referral.

I believe that both these types of decision, and the criteria by which they are made, can be made explicit. Once they are made explicit we can assess the criteria, debate or validate them. But how do we make a decision procedure explicit?

Any process can be viewed as a function that "maps" from a domain of definition to a range of values. Decision processes can therefore be regarded as functions for mapping from situations to actions. Different types of decision are formulated as different functions. In a knowledge-based approach one way of doing this is to include within the knowledge base information which specifies the domain, range and the rules for each decision. For example, the diagnosis of dyspepsia might be represented diagrammatically along the lines illustrated in Figure 3.

This illustrates one view of the management of the patient. If the "possible-cause" rules suggest that an organic condition may be responsible for the dyspepsia, then the decision may be taken to attempt a differential diagnosis, by attempting to establish facts which will differentiate, verify or eliminate the various alternatives. Each of these decisions can now be formulated as explicit functions, as illustrated in Figure 4.

TOWARDS A REPRESENTATION OF PRIMARY CARE POLICY

If it is accepted that we can formulate decisions in this explicit way, a very much more radical possibility is now before us, one which is at the core of the general practitioner's work. We have passed too quickly over the decision to embark on a differential diagnosis. In the rule given (rule 3) we are really stating a general policy, albeit

```
┌─────────────────────────────────────────────────────────────┐
│                    DYSPEPSIA (HISTORY)                      │
│                   ╱      │      ╲                           │
│                  ╱  possible causes                         │
│                 ╱        │        ╲                         │
│         Gastric cancer  Peptic ulcer   Cholecystitis        │
│                         ╱      ╲                            │
│                       D.U.     G.U.                         │
└─────────────────────────────────────────────────────────────┘
                              ↓
┌─────────────────────────────────────────────────────────────┐
│                    diagnosis decision                       │
└─────────────────────────────────────────────────────────────┘
                              ↓
┌─────────────────────────────────────────────────────────────┐
│                        DIAGNOSIS                            │
│                   ╱        ↑       ╲                        │
│        Differentiation   Verification   Elimination         │
│           rules             rules           rules           │
└─────────────────────────────────────────────────────────────┘
```

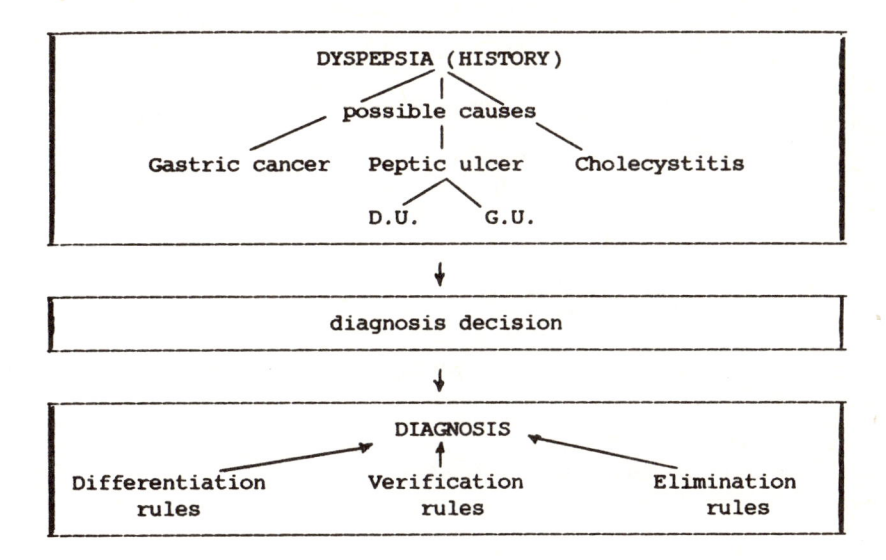

FIGURE 3

An illustrative view of part of the decision network for dyspepsia. Particular patterns in the history suggest possible organic causes. If it is decided to attempt a differential diagnosis then various types of rules can be used to distinguish, verify or eliminate alternative diagnoses.

a very simple one. The policy is not really limited to dyspepsia, it might be better to generalise it. For example, "if any problem could be caused by some organic condition that could be treated by the GP then it may be appropriate to attempt a differential diagnosis". (I have assumed that a differential diagnosis is probably inappropriate when a problem is thought to be functional or psychological in origin). Rules may also be formulated for other kinds of decision that the GP considers necessary. Contingencies may arise which indicate that action should be postponed, or that the patient should be referred, or that no action should be taken. It is desirable that the basis of such judgments be made explicit wherever possible. Brooke et al. (1983) suggest that the GP has a "cognitive map" of decisions. We might represent a cognitive map of the major classes of primary care decisions as a network, as in Figure 5. The arrows in the network summarise how the decisions are interrelated. An assessment of risk will depend upon decisions about the history, or decisions about possible diagnoses, for example.

```
Decision     possible cause of dyspepsia
Domain       {gi-signs}
Range        peptic-ulcer, gastric-cancer, gall-stones, ... functional
Function
    1.   If Patient is elderly, and
            Patient has-symptom recent-weight-loss
         then gastric-cancer is-a-possible-cause-of dyspepsia,

    2.   If Patient has-symptom pain, and
            pain has-location right-hypochondrium, and
            pain has-severity severe, or
            pain has-pattern occasional-attacks
         then cholecystitis is-a-possible-cause-of dyspepsia,
         etc
```

```
Decision  Attempt a differential diagnosis of dyspepsia
Domain    {possible-causes-of-dyspepsia}
Range     Differential-diagnosis-of-dyspepsia
Function
    3.   If Condition is-a-possible-cause-of dyspepsia, and
            Condition is-a locally-treatable-condition
         then decide differential-diagnosis-of dyspepsia
         etc.
```

```
Decision  Differential diagnosis of dyspepsia
Domain    {possible-causes-of-dyspepsia}
Range     duodenal-ulcer, gastric-ulcer, gastric-cancer, ... gall-stones
Function
    4.   If peptic-ulcer is-a-possible-cause-of dyspepsia, and
            pain is-aggravated-by food, and
            pain is-immediately-after meals
         then gastric-ulcer is-a-possible-cause-of dyspepsia
         etc.
```

FIGURE 4

Decisions are viewed as complex functions which link situations with possible conclusions or actions. These functions can then be viewed as networks of possible decisions. The decisions in figure 3 are formulated, hypothetically, as a number of IF ... THEN ... decision rules.

We must provide content as well as form in such a model of primary care decision-making however. It is my belief that many, perhaps all, of the criteria for the general classes of decision depicted in Figure 5 can be represented in terms of rules. Rules can represent a GP's subjective, even personal, policy on these questions. However, in order to formulate such policies so that a computer can follow them or just to explicate the logic behind them, we need to extend our rule machinery a little.

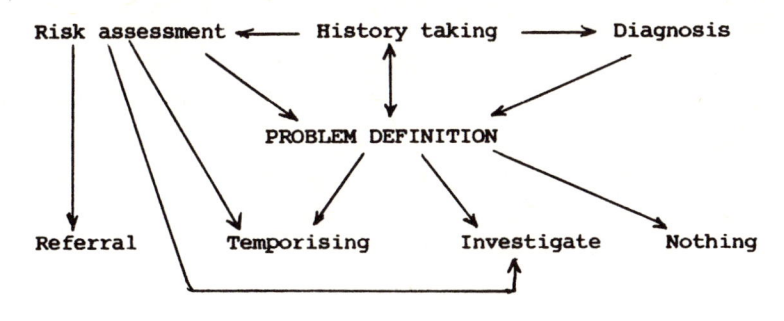

```
Risk assessment ←—— History taking ——→ Diagnosis
         ↘           ↓            ↙
            PROBLEM DEFINITION
         ↙         ↓     ↘         ↘
Referral    Temporising   Investigate   Nothing
```

FIGURE 5

Many types of decision made by GPs are general, "policy" decisions which subsume particular decisions for particular medical problems. These policy decisions can also be viewed as a network.

Rules like those in Figure 4 are primarily "special case rules", they specify particular symptoms, signs and patterns which may occur in a patient history of dyspepsia. Special case rules have the disadvantage, however, that they can only be applied in exactly specified conditions - special cases. Consequently knowledge bases containing purely special case rules may have to be very large to cover all possible situations. Also such systems are brittle; if a new situation is encountered, even if it only differs in detail from those covered by the rules, then the problem falls outside the area of competence of the system. A better way of expressing knowledge is in the form of generalised rules which can cover many specific situations, including many which may not have been foreseen in detail by the system designers. One kind of general rule is obtained by substituting variables for some or all of the objects mentioned in the rule.

For example, consider the referral decision which we might characterise as "the problem of referring all and only those patients who should be referred". A possible referral policy, covering some easily recognisable situations is formulated as an explicit set of rules in Figure 6.

THE VALIDITY OF POLICIES

Not everyone will agree with these rules. However, the very fact that they can be questioned is a considerable strength. All medical technology embodies design decisions, often with clinical implications. Even the definition of and justification for something as simple as a normal range is usually unavailable to the GP and can cause confusion when a value is marginal. The intelligibility of the rules in Figure 6 is in strong contrast. Consequently the technology is open to

```
Decision     referral
Domain       {patients}, {problems}, {diseases}
Range        {patients}, {specialists}
Function
```

4. If **Patient** is-suspected-of **Disease**, and
    Disease is-a-kind-of progressive-disease, and
    (**Disease** is-associated-with high-morbidity, or
    Disease is-associated-with high-mortality), and
    Specialist is-a-specialist-in **Disease**
   then **Patient** should-be-referred-to **Specialist**

5. If **Problem** is-a-problem-for **Patient**, and
    Problem could-be-caused-by **Disease**, and
    Disease is-a-kind-of life-threatening-condition, and
    Patient is-anxious-about **Disease**, and
    Specialist is-a-specialist-in **Disease**
   then **Patient** should-be-referred-to **Specialist**

6. If **Problem** is-a-problem-for **Patient**, and
    Problem is-a long-standing-problem, and
    Problem is-inconvenient-for **Patient**, and
    Specialist is-a-specialist-in **Disease**
   then **Patient** should-be-referred-to **Specialist**

FIGURE 6

Policy decisions can also be formulated as rules. However, the rules are not "special-case rules" and do not refer explicitly to particular kinds of disease, patient etc. They include variables (in bold) so that they refer to classes of event rather than particular events.

professional scrutiny and it is possible to debate the validity of the policy embodied in the rules.

The policy can be examined from three points of view:

1. Is the policy consistent?

2. Does it cover enough situations - is it complete?

3. Does it prescribe the right actions in the right circumstances - is it correct?

By formulating the policy as rules we obtain benefits in all these areas. Although the rules use familiar terms they are, from a formal standpoint, logical formulae which are sufficiently simple that some kinds of logical consistency can be checked. A trivial example is that of finding simple contradictions, as when two rules with the same conditions (IF.....) make different conclusions (THEN.....).

We can never be sure that a policy is complete and covers all possible contingencies. Sometimes, however, we can detect that it is incomplete. If a policy is just a special sort of function which relates contingencies to actions then, once the range of possible contingencies, or the domain of possible actions has been specified, it is possible to see if the rules of the policy fail to mention any of the contingencies or actions.

The hardest question of all is the one of how we judge a policy to be correct. The problem is not new. For years medical decision theorists have captured "rational" policies for treatment selection, resource utilisation, and so on, by combining measures of outcome likelihood with estimates of subjective utility, using various mathematical procedures. It is my belief that rules can express our intuitions about desirable policies more naturally than mathematical procedures. Rules allow us to express arbitrary concepts and relationships, not just numerical ones. Rules, furthermore, appear to be a common way of expressing written policies (as in legislation and regulations) which suggests that they express our intuitions fairly directly. For a patient-centred GP the validity of a policy for referral, or anything else, is determined by the extent to which the outcomes of that policy agree with his intuitions about whether that patient should be referred. Often there is no other practical standard.

It must be acknowledged, of course, that individual intuitions may be controversial. But the argument holds if we talk about trying to arrive at a consensus policy, rather than a correct one. Arriving at a consensus about policy depends upon the community being able to discuss its options in a common language. Once again the key is the intelligibility that rules seem to offer as a language for expressing decision criteria.

Finally, I think that many of these remarks about knowledge, rules and policies are useful, quite apart from the desirability or acceptability of decision technology in general practice. They are primarily about being articulate and logical. Even if the rules never find their way into a computer, the process of thrashing out a reasonably consistent, complete and explicit consensus on the criteria of medical judgment will surely be helpful and refreshing.

REFERENCES

Brooke, J. B., Rector, A. L., Sheldon, M. G. (1984). A Review of Studies of Decision-Making in General Practice. Medical Informatics, 9, 45-53.

Brooke, J. B., Rector, A. L., Sheldon, M. G., Langham, A. (1985). Doctors' Perceptions of Problems in Clinical Decision-Making in General Practice. Unpublished research report, Department of Community Health, University of Nottingham.

Duda, R. O. and Shortliffe, E. H. (1983). "Expert Systems Research," Science.

Fox, J. (1983). Formal and Knowledge-Based Methods in Decision Technology. Invited review paper for the proceedings of the 9th Research Conference on Subjective Probability, Utility and Decision-Making. Groningen, The Netherlands.

Fox, J. and Alvey, P. A. (1983), Computer Assisted Medical Decision-Making. British Medical Journal, 287,

Fox, J. and Rector, A. (1982). Expert Systems for Primary Medical Care. Automedica, 4, 123-130.

Spiegelhalter, D. J. and Knill-Jones, R. P. (1984). Statistical and knowledge-based approaches to clinical decision-support systems, with an application in gastroenterology. J. Roy. Statist. Soc., A 147, part 1, pp 35-77

11
Implications of Research on Clinical Decision-making for the Design of Decision Support Systems

A.L. Rector and D.C. Dodson

INTRODUCTION

The greatest difficulties in designing decision support systems for general practice are in deciding what the system should do and what factors it should take into account. What functions will actually be useful to doctors? What functions will doctors actually use? What are the factors which doctors actually take into account in making decisions?

The history of computers in medicine has too often been one of much technical accomplishment but little clinical application (Friedman and Gustafson, 1977). Some of the problem has, until recently, been the equipment which has been clumsy and expensive. However, what is more important is that doctors have not perceived the systems to be of sufficient value to warrant either their trouble or their expense. If the potential of the new generation of decision support systems is not to be lost in the same way, we need to have the answers to a number of important questions about how doctors make decisions and how information systems might complement their skills (Fox and Rector, 1982). Providing this knowledge is an important task for researchers in medical decision-making.

One task is to provide the information on which to base the choice of strategies for decision support systems from amongst the choices advocated by different centres. A second is to answer a group of questions which are important in implementing a system regardless of their basic strategy - for instance: What are the criteria for decisions? What are the basic concepts used by doctors in practice? What level of detail gives the best results?

CURRENT MODELS FOR DECISION SUPPORT SYSTEMS

There are several different models for decision support systems currently advocated by different centres. The 'traditional' system is essentially a robot consultant to whom the doctor goes for advice when confronted with a difficult case. Mycin (Shortliffe, 1976) fits this category as do Internist (Pople, 1982) and Casnet/Expert (Kulikowski and Weiss, 1982). Each of these systems provides one best suggestion as to the diagnosis and/or treatment for the patient.

This model assumes that the doctor can best be helped by being offered global advice on the decision as a whole. No theory of medical decision-making is necessary as the system functions autonomously. How the doctor would have approached the problem is important in designing explanation facilities and perhaps in controlling the order in which questions are asked. However, the decision is independent of considerations of the nature of any deficiencies in the doctor's own decision-making. It is perhaps worth noting that this model has not generally been received with wild enthusiasm by the medical profession.

Other approaches seek to aid in specific aspects of decision-making and supplement specific potential weaknesses in human performance. Although most systems make use of a mix of strategies, it is useful conceptually to consider five main functions:

- Extending the range of possibilities considered.

- Extending and systematising past experience.

- Providing general medical information.

- Checking for possible slips and omissions.

- Improving the reliability and accuracy of analysis of information gathered.

In addition, it is useful to break systems down along another axis into two groups:

- Those which the doctor consults when he is aware that he has a problem.

- Those which are activated spontaneously in response to some specific patient problem or possible error on the part of the doctor.

Examples of systems using various combinations of these strategies exist, but no general theory is available to help system designers select the best mix of functions for different applications. The following sections consider each of these functions in more detail and suggest avenues for research relevant to each.

EXTENDING THE RANGE OF POSSIBILITIES

One of the most consistent findings of the studies of doctors' decision-making is that doctors tend to narrow the range of possibilities considered early in the decision-making process. It appears that they are often reluctant to widen it again even if the fact or information which makes the original choice highly unlikely. (Brooke and Sheldon 1985; Brooke, Rector and Sheldon, 1984).

One potential function of an information system is to attempt to guard against this tendency. In its simplest form, one might provide merely an automated form of the standard references on differential diagnosis and management. The most obvious problem is that such a system would tend to flood doctors with more information than can be used effectively. The indexing of the manual versions is necessarily coarse and the information provided exhaustive. The fact that systems of this type are not in widespread use may reflect scepticism on the part of the profession about their usefulness.

However, a computer assisted system need not suffer from the same problems as a manual system. It should be possible to design a system which would provide a list tailored to the individual patient of likely diagnoses or treatments. The costs of extending the system in this way are twofold. The computer system would be much more complicated, edging into the area of 'expert systems'. The computer system would also need to be given more information about the patient. Either the doctor would have to enter more information or the system would need to get access to the information in some other way - e.g. via an automated medical record or patient interviewing system.

A system built along these lines would behave markedly differently from the 'traditional' consulting systems and would have to be evaluated differently. The test would be not whether it got the diagnosis or treatment 'correct' but whether it mentioned all the important possibilities while still being sufficiently selective to be useful. It must be useful in the situations in which such problems actually occur, including cases of multiple disease. Relatively little information is available about which common diseases tend to coexist in the same patients and which combinations of presentations are troublesome. For instance, recent work in this unit suggests that abdominal complaints relatively rarely cause 'decision-making problems' when they present alone, but frequently do so when they are complicated by some other coexisting condition.

Alternatively, this approach may be more valuable as an adjunct to other strategies. The ability of statistically-based systems to select very accurately amongst a limited number of alternatives may need to be supplemented before it is satisfactory for general clinical use. Paradoxically, in order to achieve accuracy in discriminating amongst diagnoses, the range of diagnoses considered is often restricted so as to include only the more common causes of the complaint. Although this often leads to much better average performance than that achieved previously by the doctors unaided, it provides no help with cases which lie outside the limited range covered. A different method of providing suggestions as to unusual diagnoses is needed. One example of an existing system which has gone some way in this direction is the system for the diagnosis of the acute abdomen developed by de Dombal at Leeds. After the most probable diagnoses are given it can provide an additional list of rare conditions which can produce similar presentations.

What is the optimal amount of information to give the doctor? How should the 'significant' information be selected? How many alternatives should be given? How should the doctor control what information is provided? How much information should the doctor be asked to provide? What sorts of information?

Is this approach more important in difficult cases where the doctor is puzzled or in a common symptom where the presentation of an unusual cause for a common complaint may be missed? If suggestions are to be offered spontaneously by the system, what sort of danger signals should trigger them?

EXTENDING DOCTORS' EXPERIENCE

Much of a doctor's decision-making is ultimately based on his own personal experience. The range of experience which any one doctor can collect and use effectively is limited both by the cases he sees and the scope of his memory. Several centres have concentrated on providing doctors with a means of extending the ability to recall 'similar' cases, both to help doctors make better use of their own experience and to help them to pool experience. Two of the best known are the Duke University Cardiology system and the AEDM system at Rennes in France (Lenoir and Chales, 1980). A new system from Emory University, Atlanta, Georgia (Camp et al., 1983) which is integrated into the hospital information system has been reported recently.

Each of these systems allows doctors to review previous 'similar' cases efficiently. The criteria for what constitutes a 'similar' case can be varied to produce a manageable number of cases and to explore different aspects of the current problem. The diagnosis, management and outcome of the previous cases can be reviewed and tabulated in a variety of ways in order to help the doctor evaluate the most appropriate approach to the present case. Such systems have the potential to make the experience of specialised centres widely available to the profession as a whole.

Several related questions arise: How should the information be summarised so that it can be absorbed? Is this actually an effective way of helping the doctor make decisions? Will it, for instance, widen doctors' range of consideration or will it be used so selectively as merely to confirm prior unconscious preconceptions. How can the designers of such a system ensure that it is used effectively? What are the most important categories? What are the questions which really need to be asked? Can the information to answer them be recorded routinely?

GENERAL MEDICAL INFORMATION

There are of course many systems which have been developed to provide other sorts of general medical information. Most aim to provide easier access to information contained in standard reference works. Systems, particularly on pharmacology and therapeutics, are becoming available. It remains to be seen whether or not in practice they will be sufficiently more convenient than their manual counterparts to gain wide acceptance in the profession. Certainly, the systems provided to date on British Telecom's Prestel service have made much less impact than had originally been hoped. It will be extremely interesting to follow the fate of the new services being offered by AMANet and the various commercial vendors of this type of service. When the problems of access to the hardware to deliver the systems are overcome, it may prove that these are fully as valuable as any of the more sophisticated systems.

ACCIDENTAL SLIPS AND OMISSIONS

Before the doctor can benefit from the systems described above, he must be aware that there is a problem. However, many of the problems in medical care occur precisely because the doctor is not aware that a problem exists.

Doctors frequently make slips or omissions in routine care. This has been documented by every study which has attempted to audit the care of common chronic diseases. In perhaps the best known series of such studies, McDonald (1976) showed that these errors were unrelated to the level of training of the doctors involved, and he attributed them to information overload. More recently the work of Reason and Mycielska (1982) may provide a more convenient paradigm of the causes of 'absent minded' slips. It suggests that they are probably inevitable in any task which becomes routine, particularly if attention is required to transfer rapidly among several different activities. In effect, such errors are seen as the cost we pay for our skills.

One of the possible functions for a computer system is to monitor for such errors. To do so we need adequate information on the criteria for various actions. Alarms which are rung too frequently or are too often spurious are soon ignored. A careful analysis of doctor's tasks and routines might be able to pinpoint the likely danger areas. Combined with sensible consideration of the medical importance of various tasks, it should help to provide a system which is seen as helpful rather than a nuisance.

A more attractive solution is to use an information system to structure doctors' tasks so that they are less prone to slips. One might hope that the problem would be helped by an information system which helped to make clear the structure of the tasks to be accomplished and to identify those which were still outstanding. Any features in the information system which serve to help bring the attention back to critical areas should be helpful.

This suggests integrating the decision support system into the medical record system. The presentation of the manual medical record system is dictated by the needs of data entry - the only thing which is practical with a paper record is to record items serially or at most a few sections. Reorganising the record once it is created is difficult if not impossible. To date, most computer based medical record systems have been fundamentally little different from the manual systems they replaced.

Recently a few centres have begun to integrate the decision support systems into record systems. In the long term, this suggests the possibility of record systems which could be, at least to some degree, self-organising. The presentation of the record could, therefore, be designed primarily to aid the doctor in retrieving information and, more importantly, in recognising the tasks which need to be performed. The most widely publicised system of this type is the Oncocyn system being developed at Stanford for the treatment of patients on cancer chemotherapy protocols. In this area the model of the process of care is provided by the protocols.

Developing such a system in a much more varied area of medicine such as general practice requires a clear model of the way in which doctors conceptualise medical tasks. What are the tasks implied by different patient problems? How do they interrelate? Can any of them be done automatically?

These questions must form part of a broader enquiry into the practical protocols for patient care. There must be a way of representing to the system not only the bare medical facts, but also their relative importance. It must, for instance, be possible to indicate that all patients on diuretics should have their potassium monitored, but that this is particularly important in patients who are also on digitalis.

Coupled with this, there needs to be an investigation of how different presentations affect the way doctors perform their tasks. Can we show that different presentations actually do affect their liability to 'slips'?

CRITIQUING

A separate approach has recently been suggested by Miller (1983). Rather than asking the system for suggestions per se, the doctor enters a suggested plan of action and the information system provides a commentary on the plan. The system seems to offer a number of advantages. Doctors report liking the system. The system takes in only the information which is supplied - and that in free text format. The doctor is not asked to work through a long questionnaire session at the keyboard. The information which is supplied is directed at the decisions which the doctor has made (or failed to make).

The system as it is currently used includes sophisticated natural language interfaces for both input and output, and is consulted as a separate activity. However, the idea of building such a facility into a general medical record package seems highly attractive as a long term goal, provided that we can be convinced that doctors really will find it useful.

IMPROVING THE ANALYSIS OF THE INFORMATION GATHERED

Improvements in the accuracy of the analysis of information gathered is what occurs to people first when they think of 'computer aided decision-making'. It has frequently been shown that statistical procedures can improve the diagnosis of a variety of conditions, and in addition a number of systems based on artificial intelligence have been developed which give advice aimed at improving diagnosis and management.

Different approaches to computer aids for decision-making address different aspects of the analysis problem and require different information. Unless specially trained, people have been shown to combine probabilities inefficiently and inaccurately. Statistical systems correct for these errors and have been highly effective in a number of situations. If failures of this type are the cause of error, then this would appear to be the technique of choice. The structure of the decision and the manner of the interrelations amongst items are relatively unimportant.

Systems based on artificial intelligence techniques tend to emphasise the richness of this overall structure and these interrelations, and use this to compensate for limited numerical accuracy. It is hoped that they will be able to deal with situations where numerical information is lacking or irrelevant. However, not only are formal methods in this area still in their infancy by comparison with statistics, but the methods for obtaining the relevant concepts are still ad hoc. Much more work is needed.

The other major area of analytic techniques is formal decision analysis which seeks to use statistical methods not only to discriminate amongst diagnoses, but to select among alternative actions. They depend crucially on estimates of the 'utilities' of each outcome. In some areas of acute illness it may, at least, be relatively clear what the dimensions should be - length of survival, severe pain etc. In many situations in general practice even this information is currently lacking, and the researcher seeking to apply them finds himself in much the same position as the worker in artificial intelligence, seeking to define the basic concepts and criteria which are relevant.

MEDICAL CONCEPTS, EXPLANATIONS, INTERFACE AND MEDICAL SIGNIFICANCE

Regardless of the basic strategy chosen, the designer of a decision support system must decide how to organise information, what items to include, and how the interface with the doctor is to be organised. These are fundamental questions which will have as much to do with the success of the system as the model chosen. The structure chosen must capture the medical significance of the situation faithfully. They should approach doctors using the natural level of detail which the doctors would themselves use.

Discovering the basic way in which doctors conceptualise a problem and the criteria which are actually relevant to general practice decisions is by no means straightforward. In the few studies done by this unit, we have found repeatedly that the information which we are given initially in the abstract bears little resemblance to what is actually done in practice. Much to the investigators' discomfiture, every patient appears to be a special case. The factors which actually influence therapy must be a major task for research decision-making. While many books make generalisations about the factors which are, or ought to be, taken into account in primary care, studies which show what is actually done are very difficult to find.

Producing a satisfactory explanation for decisions depends on recognising what were the most significant factors in the decision. The work on systems which is based on artificial intelligence places particular emphasis on the ability of the systems to explain their actions. The entire thrust of the work on 'critiquing' is based on the idea of explanation. However, if it is to be satisfactory in primary care, the system must be based on the criteria which are used by doctors in practice in the field.

The problem of the 'man machine interface' with doctors goes far beyond the mechanical questions such as whether to use a light pen, 'mouse', or traditional keyboard, important though these are to any particular system. The concepts used in the system and the way they are presented must match the users' needs. Systems which demand that they be given information in much more detail than the doctor would normally use to a colleague or which have their own idiosyncratic definitions and concepts are unlikely to gain widespread acceptance.

Computer designers have tended to blame users who are impatient with the detailed entry the designers have demanded. Perhaps a richer approach with more global concepts and many more features which are 'understood' unless explicitly contradicted would be more appropriate. If doctors do make many of their decisions on the basis of global patterns, ought not this to be the way in which the information is captured?

This question, sometimes referred to in other concepts as the 'chunk size', has been little investigated by researchers in clinical decision-making. What is the basic level of detail at which doctors usually manipulate concepts? How much does it vary between doctors? How much with different situations? Can we design systems which operate effectively nearer to the doctors' usual level of conceptual 'chunking' without sacrificing the accuracy and rigour needed? Might we even improve them by gaining more widespread support?

CONCLUSION

Decision support systems for clinical practice are in their infancy. The development of new software and hardware gives the possibility for radically new and different approaches to supporting and extending doctors' work, to the benefit of both doctors and patients. Currently the search for new methods of using systems and the process of designing systems for different clinical problems are entirely empirical. Systematic development of alternatives is hampered by the lack of any coherent theory of medical decision-making, particularly any theory which takes into account the range of activities in general practice.

Work is needed to help to identify the areas with the greatest payoff and the most acceptable strategies. How the elements of doctors' decision-making strategies affect their interaction with potential systems also need to be investigated in order to produce congenial systems. Our success in applying new techniques will depend on how well these questions are answered.

Acknowledgements

This work was supported in part by a grant from the Medical Research Council.

REFERENCES

Brooke, J. B., & Sheldon, M.G., (1985). Decision = Patient with Problem + Doctor with Problem. This volume.

Brooke, J. B., Rector, A. L. and Sheldon, M. G., (1984) A Review of Studies of Decision-making in General Practice. Medical Informatics, 9: 45-53.

Camp, H. N., Ridley, M. L. and Walker, H. K., (1983), Theresa: A Computerised Medical Consultant based on the Patient Record. In: M. J. Ball and O. Wigertz (Eds.) Proceedings of MEDINFO 83, Amsterdam, North Holland, pp. 612-617.

Friedman, R. E. and Gustafson, D. H., (1977) Computers in Medicine: A Critical Review. Computers in Biomedical Research, 10, pp. 199-204.

Fox, J. and Rector, A. L., (1982) Expert Systems for the G.P.? Automedica, 4, 123-130.

Kulikowski, C. A. and Weiss, S. M., (1982) Representation of Expert Knowledge for Consulation: The CASNET and EXPERT Projects, in P. Szolovits (Ed.) Artificial Intelligence in Medicine, Boulder, Colorado, Westview Press/AAAS, pp. 21-56.

Lenoir, P. and Chales, G. (1980) Pourquoi et comment aider les medecinsa porter les diagnostics. Medical Informatics, 5, 4, pp. 281-289.

McDonald, C.J. (1976) Protocol based computer reminders; the quality of care and the non-perfectability of man. New England Journal of Medicine, 295, pp.1351-1355.

Miller, Perry L. (1983) Critiquing anesthetic management: the 'Attending' computer system. Anesthesiology, 58, pp.362-369.

Miller, Perry L. (1984) Attending: critiquing a physician's management plan. IEEE Transactions on Pattern Analysis and Machine Intelligence, Vol. PAMI-5, pp.449-461.

Miller, Perry L., and Black, Henry R. (1984) Medical plan-analysis by computer: critiquing the pharmacologic management of essential hypertension. Computers and Biomedical Research, 17, pp.38-54.

Pople, H. E. Jr. (1982) Heuristic Methods for Imposing Structure on Il l Structured Problems: The Structuring of Medical Diagnostics,' in P. Szolovits (Ed.) Artificial Intelligence in Medicine, Boulder, Colorado, Westview Press/AAAS, pp. 119-190.

Reason, J. and Mycielska, K. (1982) Absent-Minded? The Psychology of Mental Lapses and Everyday Errors, Englewood Cliffs, N.J., Prentice Hall.

Shortliffe, E. H. (1976), Computer-Based Medical Consultations: MYCIN, New York, Elsevier/North Holland.

12
Factors Influencing Referrals by General Practitioners to Consultants

B.J.M. Aulbers

Nothing is easier than to philosophize about a common topic about which little is known. For every general practitioner, referring patients to medical specialists is a common event. But referring patients is like driving a car: we handle it daily, but we have no knowledge of the mechanism. Quite a lot has been published about the numbers and costs of referrals, differences in the methods of general practitioners and specialists, communications between the two and, more especially, the lack of them, but virtually nothing is to be found on the question why a general practititioner refers a particular patient to a specialist. The obvious answer is: because he considers it necessary. However, according to George Bernard Shaw no question is as difficult to answer as a question to which the answer is obvious.

For this Workshop we can pose the central question: Why does this general practitioner refer this patient to a consultant now? Further on: Why does he refer to this consultant? Which factors can influence the decision?

Publications about referrals in different countries are not comparable, because of the different health systems, Conditions for referrals may be different for patients, general practitioners and consultants in different countries. The literature on referrals agrees in three respects:

- the aim of a referral has to be to get a useful effect;

- everywhere the costs of consequences from referrals have increased strongly in the last decades;

- strikingly large differences have been found in the number of referrals between general practitioners.

A referral can have a useful effect for the patient, for the doctor or for both. The useful effect may consist of:

- treatment, reassurance or "second opinion" for the patient

- diagnosis or reassurance for the doctor or to get rid of the patient for some time.

According to various authors, strikingly large differences have been found in the number of referrals by general practitioners. For example, Goss (1982) in Britain reports a variation of 0.5-15 referrals for 100 patient consultations. In the Netherlands the association of sick-funds reports for 1979 a variation of 218-766 referrals for 1000 subscribing members.

Everywhere the costs of referrals have increased sharply during the last 10-20 years. Referrals bring patients from fairly simple and cheap health provision to a more complicated and expensive one. An increasing number of consultants have at their disposal an increasing number of tools for diagnosis and treatment in their clinics and out-patient departments.

These large differences in the number of referrals by general practitioners can be partly explained by population factors such as number of patients, their age, sex and social class, or influence of ethnic minorities, and also partly by factors related to the practice, such as location and distance from a hospital. Even when these things are taken into account, however, it is still found that one general practitioner has a higher referral rate than another.

O'Cummins, Jarman and White (1981) have studied these individual differences in their own practice in Westminster. They speak of differences in 'referral thresholds', which they define as 'the level at which the stimulus of a consultation produces a referral'. These differences were found to persist even after their practices had been standardized in terms of age, sex and social class.

Recently the Dutch Institute for General Practice published the results of our enquiry into the referrals of 806 general practitioners, working in single-handed practices, (Dopheide, 1982). According to this publication the number of referrals by these practitioners are influenced by a number of factors like:

- a smaller distance from the surgery to an outpatient department or hospital, and more facilities available lead to more referrals;

- a greater number of old people leads to more referrals, but not for all specialities;

- regional factors: in the Southern part of the Netherlands more patients are referred to consultants;

- when the general practitioner has a broad conception of his task, he will refer a smaller number of his patients to consultants; this has more influence in small practices;

- in this enquiry there was no influence of the years of experience or the age of the practitioners - there was no influence of the workload of the doctor.

In contrast to these findings Morrell, Gage and Robinson (1971) report that older doctors do not refer as many patients as younger ones: "They tend to be more tolerant of diagnostic uncertainty than younger doctors".

We have to consider these conclusions cautiously, because some factors are interdependent and terms like workload, social structure of the practice and even referral do not have the same definition in different populations. Moreover the Netherlands have a quite unique health-system in the world, although it may be compared in many aspects with the British health-system.

In Wisconsin, U.S.A., Ludke (1982) carried out a study of the factors which can influence the decision to refer. Thirty-eight doctors, most of them primary care physicians, were presented with a list of factors and asked to put them in order of importance in their own opinion. The factors had been drawn up and defined beforehand and all related to rational considerations.

According to this study the chief factors in the decision whether or not to refer and in the decision as to which specialist were:

- quality of patient management;

- patients' results;

- individual patient management and care;

- habits of neighbouring colleagues.

Ludke's study is not unconditionally relevant to the countries around the North Sea, because it is based on circumstances in the U.S.A. It is however, indicative (though in my view too one-sidedly) of rational factors. Irrational and emotional factors undoubtedly play a part in the referral process, but are difficult to bring to light.

In Britain Goss (1982) reports a smaller number of referrals when the general practitioner has more years of experience, but a greater number when he has more knowledge in a particular branch himself. He cites these observations in favour of a move away from simple ratewatching and towards an evaluation of the appropriateness of the individual episode of referral.

In this respect Bourne's study from the Tavistock Clinic London (Bourne,1976) seems to vindicate this more personal approach. Using a Balint group a number of general trends were observed as well as some individual peculiarities. Referral could be used both to keep and to reject patients. The choice of consultant could be helpful or deliberately punitive. Patients seen as 'on the fringe' (e.g. transients, recent arrivals, temporary residents, etc.) were more likely to be referred. Some referrals seemed to contribute more to the development of the relationship between the general practitioner and the consultant than to the care of the patient; also the doctor's own dependency needs could be fulfilled by a referral. Perhaps most strikingly, examples were found of specific illness phobias among doctors resulting in inappropriate referral. According to Bourne, doctors in general have a particular and often quite conscious horror of specific illness, different for each doctor.

I shall attempt to throw some light on a number of factors which can play a part in referral decisions. I shall also endeavour to indicate some possibilities for further research in this area. In working out these ideas I shall confine myself to the Dutch health-system and to primary referrals. By this I mean referrals resulting from consultation between the general practitioner and the patient and relating to an episode of sickness or abnormality for which there has been no previous referral.

In a primary referral the initiative usually comes from the general practitioner, the patient or the two together.

A referral decision can be broken down into:

- the decision whether or not to refer;

- if referral is decided upon, the decision as to which specialist.

As factors which can play a part in the decision for or against referral I can mention practice-related, doctor-related and patient-related factors.

Factors Influencing Referrals by GPs to Consultants

1. Practice-related factors:

    - Town or country: no influence as such;

    - Availability of specialist facilities: the closer the hospital is and the more specialist facilities there are, the more referrals will be made;

    - Population factors: the number of referrals increase with age (but not for all specialities);

    - Habits of neighbouring colleagues (Ludke, 1982)

2. Doctor-related factors:

    - The doctor's work load seems to have no influence;

    - Reasons for referral: these can be divided into the classic triad - diagnosis, treatment and reassurance, with all their possible combinations.

    The factors relevant to these reasons for referral are as follows:

    (a) In the case of a request for treatment:

    - diagnosis or suspicion of a serious disorder;

    - the disorder can be treated better by the specialist;

    - the specialist will be more able to deal with possible complications.

    (b) In the case of a request for consultation:

    - the diagnosis is uncertain and the uncertainty cannot be diminished without specialist consultation;

    Two situations can be distinguished here:

    - a high probability of a serious disorder;

    - the disorder is probably not serious, but the consequences of assessing whether a particular disease is present or not, are serious

- unexpected complications in what at first appeared to be a minor disorder;

- vague complaints whose causes are not clear. There is more chance of referral for complaints of this kind (Does, 1979).

(c) In the case of reassurance:

- number of years experience: there are different opinions about the influence of this factor;

- own research or not: depending on personal enthusiasm, involvement or the feeling of being at home in this field (Goss, 1982);

- fear of missing serious diseases: this fear is partly produced by the general practitioner's chiefly clinical training in which certain diagnostic errors are regarded as blunders;

- fear of failure: doctors with high figures for supplementary X-ray or laboratory examinations often have high referral figures (Does, 1979)

- fear of legal consequences: the increase in lawsuits can cause a general practitioner to refer patients more often, for safety;

- fear of medicalization of the problem or of fixation on his complaints on the part of the patient can deter a general practitioner from referral.

Besides these rational factors, irrational and negative influences can play a part in the decision for referral such as those mentioned by Bourne (1976):

- a referral could be meant to keep or to reject patients;

- the choice of consultant could be helpful or punitive;

- the doctor's own phobias or fantasies;

- inability to understand the patient or the problem;

- the doctor's lack of motivation to deal with the problem himself;

- poor communication between the doctor and the patient;
- the doctor's desire to make a good or even a bad impression on the specialist, (or on the patient);
- 'fringe' patients are more likely to be referred.

3. Patient-related factors

The initiative for referral can come from the patient himself or the decision can be arrived at jointly. According to various authors like Pel, (1975) Es and Pijlman (1970) and Carson (1982), in roughly 20% of the cases the initiative for primary referral comes from the patient.

Motives for this initiative on the part of the patient can be:

- fear of serious illness;
- fear of being 'strung along' by the general practitioner;
- lack of faith in the general practitioner's competence;
- great faith in the competence of consultants;
- 'two heads are better than one'

Financial factors are increasingly important in recent years. Realization that the public purse is not bottomless touches all aspects of health care. Referral decisions carry important considerations of cost.

No less important than the decision for or against referral is the decision as to which consultant. An important part is played here by personal factors and by previous experiences with a specialist. These factors are mentioned by Ludke (1982). They are applicable for both the general practitioner and the patient.

In my opinion, personal factors such as the GP's relationship with the consultant is one of the most important influences on the choice of the consultant. Good communications between general practitioners and clinicians are a blessing, and bad ones are a curse. On the matter of communication, a great deal has been published.

Communication is a cyclical process. A particular attitude of one person to another is often the result of previous encounters. If a specialist communicates poorly with a general practitioner the cause may very well lie in the fact that the general practitioner communicates poorly with the specialist.

What can a general practitioner expect from a referral if he gives no further explanation, provides no information and asks no questions? Communication between general practitioners and specialists is difficult enough even if all the requirements of a good referral are satisfied. The reason lies in their very different methods of problem-solving (McWhinney 1978). In the Netherlands Gerritsma and Smal (1982) investigated the problem-solving of general practitioners and clinical physicians. They used simulated patients and found a number of differences in methods used by the two groups of doctors. Remarkably, however, they found no differences in:

- attention paid to psychic and social factors;

- endeavour for completeness in gathering information;

- number of working hypotheses after the problem has been posed.

According to Gerritsma and Smal, doctors generally solve a medical problem with the help of a number of hypotheses, which they then test. In doing so, general practitioners take a more direct and specialists a more systematic approach. Both GPs and specialists generally use between three and five hypotheses.

The differences in methods can be explained by sociological factors such as differences in:

- position in the health care system;

- type of practice (alone or as part of a large unit);

- supply of patients (unselected or selected).

Gerritsma and Smal found that a notable difference exists in the behaviour of general practitioners and specialists when confronted with complications or vague, undefined complaints. Specialists evidently feel more at home with complications and can deal with them better. General practitioners have a tendency to devote more time and attention to a patient when unexpected complications arise. They 'visit' the patients more often and do more examinations or have more supplementary examinations carried out. The danger of deferring a justifiable referral is alarming.

In the case of vague, undefined complaints without complications the tendency is for the reverse to happen. General practitioners are usually content with a brief examination into somatic, psychic and social factors. Vague complaints prompt specialists to do more. They endeavour to ensure that nothing has been overlooked by carrying out the most complete possible physical, laboratory and specialist examinations. It would appear that specialists feel more at home where there are clear positive indications for a disease. General practitioners feel more at ease when a serious disease seems to be absent. According to Gerritsma and Smal, this has implications for the referral policies of general practitioners. Where there are unexpected complications they run the risk of waiting too long when referral is necessary. Conversely, referrals in cases where there are no clear indications can lead to an exhaustive examination at the second level, especially for vague complaints. The danger then is that a common abnormality will be found which is not necessarily connected with the original complaint. This can lead to referral to other specialists and somatic fixation on his complaints on the part of the patient. Attention to this danger had been drawn by Does (1979) and others.

A great deal of further research will have to be done on the extremely complex interplay between general practitioners and specialists in referrals. I believe that it is of great importance to research specific facets. Such studies can be concerned with fact gathering, the evaluation of decisions, the evaluation of correspondence and similar matters. For research on factors affecting decisions or motivation, use can be made of simulated patients, documented cases or analyses of surgery tapes. It should be realized however, that a bias is introduced in relation to reality. But perhaps one of the most simple means is to audit your own referrals for a period and discover what factors weigh most with them.

Meanwhile, the general practitioner's task as regards referrals remain unchanged. This task was excellently described in The Future General Practitioner,(1972). 'The general practitioner must in referrals to a specialist use his knowledge and skills in presenting the right patient, selecting the right specialist, explaining the referral to the first and preparing background information for the second'.

REFERENCES

Bourne, S. (1976), 'Second Opinion', Journal of the Royal College of General Practitioners, 26, 487-495.

Carson, N. E. (1982), 'The Referral Process,' Medical Journal of Australia, 1, 180-182.

Does, E. van der (1979),'Goed Verwijzen' (Good Referring), MedischContact, 34, 255-256.

Dopheide, J. P. (1982), 'Verwijzing door de huisarts' (Referrals by General Practitioner), Report Dutch Institute of General Practice, Utrecht.

Es, J. S. van and Pijlman, H. R. (1970), 'Het Verwijzen van Ziekenfonds- patienten in 122 Nederlands Huisartspraktijken' (Referring Sickfund Members in 122 Dutch General Practices), Huisarts en Wetenschap, 13, 433-449.

Gerritsma, J. G. M. and Smal, J. A. (1982), 'De Werkwijze van de Huisarts en Internist' (Working Methods of the General Practitioner and the Clinical Physician), Bunge, Utrecht.

Goss, B. M. (1982), 'Factors affecting the Decisions to Consult and the Decision to Refer,' Update, 25, 1113-1118.

Ludke, R. L. (1982), 'An Examination of the Factors that Influence Patient Referral Decision,' Medical Care, Vol. XX, No. 8, 782-796.

McWhinney, I. R. (1980) 'Decision-making in General Practice,' Journal of the Royal College of General Practitioners, Occasional Paper No. 10, 31-33.

Morrell, D. C., Gage, H. G. and Robinson, N. A. (1971), 'Referral to Hospital by General Practitioners,' Journal of the Royal College of General Practitioners, 21, 77-85.

O'Cummins, R., Jarman, B. and White, P. M. (1981), 'Do General Practitioners have Different "Referral Thresholds"?', British Medical Journal, 282. 1037-1039.

Pel, J. Z. S. (1975), 'Over de Invloed van de Huisarts op het Verwijspercentage' (On the Influence of the GP on Referring Percentage), Medisch Contact, 30, 988-990.

Royal College of General Practitioners (1972), 'The Future General Practitioner, Learning and Teaching,' London.

13
A Discussion on Aids to Decision-making in the Consultation

Mike Fitter

The session focussed on how decision-making in the consultation might be aided by decision support systems. A wide range of issues arose in a lively discussion and I have attempted to clarify some of these by imposing a structure as outlined below.

Why decision aids? The main purpose of developing aids was to improve the quality of decisions. This resulted from research which had identified 'human shortcomings' in decision-makers. These would include problems of skill level, intellect or memory capacity, and cognitive or emotional 'bias' in decision criteria. It was also recognised that there could be pressures for reducing the cost of decision-making through, for example, increasing effectiveness and speed of decisions or using paramedics in certain areas.

What areas of application? Already decision aids were successful in certain specialist areas (e.g. acute abdominal pain). Could these areas be extended to cover the range of problems dealt with by the General Practitioner?

In particular, would we ever have a system which could help the patient who complained of just feeling "tired"? Moreover, since the approach was necessarily reductive (rather than holistic), would a decision aid be compatible with a genuinely 'patient-centred' approach? Opinions differed, the optimistic view being that it was a matter of time (and hard work).

Information quality, repeatability and knowledge transfer - It was recognised that the success of a decision aid depended crucially on the accuracy of the information which was fed in, and on the agreement that could be reached by physicians on an acceptable terminology. Repeatability was the essence. However, whereas it was thought undesirable and impractical that every G.P. should have his/her own personal system 'tuned' to their own personal preferences, concern was also expressed about extracting the 'knowledge' of an individual (or small group of individuals) and establishing this as the 'norm'. This would be an unacceptable degree of standardisation. Moreover, there is not sufficient agreement on the decision goals, nor necessarily the mechanisms to reach agreement, to adopt such an approach.

Personal Policies - Whereas it might be possible in principle to develop rules which represented a 'personal policy' of a G.P. it was not clear whether this was practical or desirable. Would doctors be prepared to make all their personal policies explicit and therefore potentially public? And how would the 'rationalisation' of personal policies affect decisions?

Freezing and learning systems - Medicine is changing all the time. Diseases are disappearing and new ones arising. Is there a danger that decision support systems might 'freeze' or at least slow down new developments? It is important that changes can be planned, possibly by developing systems which can learn from experience. It was pointed out that it is not just a problem of machines being slow to change. There is a problem of how in practice rules can be modified. If new developments are built directly onto the old there is a danger of creating something akin to 'urban sprawl' which clogs many of our cities, or the cumbersome social security system which generation after generation of qualifications have made almost unworkable. There could be a danger that the whole framework of decision-making becomes too rigid; as Balint had argued, 'organising diseases is dangerous'.

The patient? How would the patients respond to decision aids? It wasn't clearly established whether improved clinical performance led to increased patient well-being, although used appropriately the decision aid could be seen as a non-invasive tool in the clinician's kit-bag. The development of patient aids designed to help patients directly, perhaps on whether to see their doctor, was thought by some to be a new and worthwhile area.

Evaluation of, and Responsibility, for Decisions - This is a crucial issue, raising the fundamental question, "what is a good decision?" An analysis of the decision process, and an assessment of the effectiveness of decisions are vital pre-conditions to the development of decision aids. When such aids exist, who is responsible for decisions made by a doctor who has passed "part or all of a decision to a decision support system" (to quote Brooke)? The doctor must be ultimately, and this emphasises how important it is that he/she understands the basis on which that decision has been made. Expert systems have the potential advantage of being able to 'explain' the rationale underlying their advice. Decisions based on mathematical models can be opaque to the decision-maker. It can be expected that there will be litigation cases in the law courts over liability for decisions made in conjunction with decision support systems. There is also a precedent suggesting negligence on the part of a physician for not using a decision aid that had been shown to be effective.

Is it inevitable? There is some feeling that these developments are in some sense inevitable; and that 'dumb' systems are irritating and 'intelligent' ones a threat. An attitude which 'glamourises' the technology and one which completely shuns it are both undesirable. In many areas of skilled work, technology has tended to turn craftsmen into technicians and create large and highly organised work units. However, Primary Care is moving in a different direction with the identification and development of specific skills combined with a more 'patient-centred' approach. It is important that the technology is harnessed to these goals.

Influencing the design - One of the most important points that emerged from the discussion was of the need for the medical profession to influence the development of decision support systems, and other technological aids. If the aids were 'person-centred' rather than 'technology-centred' they could be liberating rather than constraining. This could be to the benefit of both patients and doctors. To achieve this end the means must be established by which the profession can be the major influence in the design process. The qualities of General Practice must be identified and the decision aids designed to fit in with them. Not vice versa.

14
Developing a Unitary Model of the Clinical Management Process

Thomas R. Taylor and Michael J. Gordon

To date, in studies of clinical decision-making, most emphasis has been on the problem-solving/diagnostic phase of hospital-based practice assuming a strictly biomedical view of disease and illness. For the primary care physician a much broader biopsychosocial view of clinical decision-making is needed to cope with the early and ill-defined versions of disease and illness which we encounter and to take account of the overwhelming importance of management decision-making in primary care settings.

The research aims of our group have focused on understanding the decision-making process that underlies clinical management both from the physician's and the patient's point of view. We are particularly interested in family medicine, but have also studied general internal medicine and specialist endocrinology practice for comparative purposes. Our aim is to produce a new model of management decision-making as an aid to understanding the long-term management of diabetes. We would like to illuminate the interactive aspects of the management process and to identify areas of agreement or conflict between physician and patient so as to identify appropriate and effective interventions. These interventions will be aimed at physicians as well as patients in order to improve adherence to treatment regimens and improve both biomedical and psychosocial outcomes.

We chose diabetes mellitus as a focus for our study because it is a chronic disease with high morbidity, an unequivocal biomedical base, having a high incidence of compliance problems and a high psychosocial and economic impact on the patient and the community. It is the seventh commonest problem encountered in family practice in the United States (Kirkwood et al., 1982).

CHOICE OF METHODS

In our studies of management decision-making in diabetes mellitus, we have opted for a descriptive approach in attempting to identify the factors or issues which influence the judgement process in diabetes management. We have employed the two complementary techniques of (i) process tracing and (ii) regression based policy analysis ("policy capturing") advocated by Einhorn and Hogarth (1981). The policy analysis studies will be reported at a later date.

The process tracing approaches employed by us involves a group of techniques calling for introspection and thinking aloud by subjects. We have used two complementary types of process tracing. Our first approach was based on content analysis of verbal data from structured interview protocols. Clinicians were interviewed shortly after seeing a patient and asked to describe their approach to diabetes management in general and to that patient in particular. The aim was to identify key decisions, and cues so as to eventually infer the decision rules which underlie the management of diabetes. Our second approach used an alternative and complementary type of "process tracing" based on the use of video recordings and stimulated recall of routine visits on eight of the twenty-four physician/patient pairs used in our studies. This has provided an extra source of validation: it is discussed in detail later.

Several investigators have used process tracing techniques to describe and classify aproaches to clinical problems and tasks employed by different physicians (Elstein et al., 1978; Barrows and Abrahamson, 1964; Barrows and Bennett, 1972).

The process tracing and policy capturing techniques are regarded as complementary (Einhorn et al., 1979). The process tracing approach is an inductive approach which is used to identify key management decisions and the cues used to make them which can then be tested by deductively based policy capturing techniques. The policy capturing techniques are used to deduce the relationship between cues and decisions. Our policy capturing studies will be reported elsewhere.

The Inductive Phase: Searching for cues and decisions

(i) Process Tracing Studies of Physicians

Using a structured interview protocol developed from a review of the diabetes literature, twenty-four physicians were interviewed representing both university and community-based practices and training backgrounds in family medicine, internal medicine and endocrinology. The interviews were audio taped, transcribed and corrected by the interviewers and interviewees. Two trained analysts independently extracted all diabetes related content from the interviews in the form of first person statements. Specific wording of the statements was negotiated between the two analysts with an agreement of over 75% when the statements first extracted and over 90% on those finally chosen. This resulted in a pool of 1,496 statements (typed on index cards for further sorting) with between thirty-three and one hundred and nine statements per physician subject.

We next tried to classify the statements. They could be sorted under topic headings but they simply reproduced the topics covered in the interview structure. Our problem at this stage was lack of a coherent model of the management process. A systematic review of textbooks of clinical medicine, including clinical methods, produced only general ideas but no coherent model. An exhaustive search of the psychological and decision-making literature and of the management science literature revealed no single model which was appropriate to our needs or sufficiently well defined to allow us to train analysts to use it. Finally a single hybrid model combining concepts from the psychological and decision-making literature (Beach, 1982) and from business management literature (Mintzberg, 1973) was assembled by us, subjected to preliminary testing and analyst training and was found to hold promise. Refinements of the model (including definitions delineating critical points of transitions between the stages) eventually permitted independent judges to sort statements into the four distinct stages of our model with 86% agreement. Definitions of model stages with sample statements were submitted to a group of physicians and found clinically plausible.

The model is composed of four stages:

1. system assessment - (36% of statements for all twenty-four physicians) in which the physician constructs a picture of the diagnosis, prognosis and resources (of all kinds) available to a patient;
2. goal setting - (39%) in which the physician reconciles multiple preferences integrating these into an ordered set of goals;
3. management plan - (8%) in which a long term plan of management is chosen and
4. tactical implementation - (16%) in which the physician chooses specific actions to optimise implementation of the chosen plan and to monitor its progress.

Two percent of statements were not classified. This process of hypothesizing a model, confirming its plausibility by comprehensive and reliable sorting of statements using public definitions and establishing plausibility with practising physicians will be described in detail elsewhere.

(ii) Process Tracing Studies of Patients

The data gathering and content analysis process for patients followed exactly the same sequence as that described for physicians. Each of the twenty-four physicians provided a patient for the studies. All management related interview statements were extracted from patient transcripts by two independent analysts with interjudge agreements of 81%. The remaining statements, where there was disagreement, were resolved by negotiation to yield a total of 2,289 management related statements with fifty to one hundred and fifty-four statements per patient. There was no contact between interviewers or analysts for the patient data and those for the physician data. As with the physician data, we reviewed other available models in the health services, psychological, business management and clinical care literature before resorting to the four-stage model developed for the physicians. The Health Belief Model, Fishbein-Azjen Behavioural Intention Model and Triandis Behavioural Intention Model were all too closely linked to specific behaviours and not suitable for classifying the management related statements of chronic disease and to overall global statements and plans. We concluded that the four stage model provided the best vehicle for comprehensive understanding of the managment picture from the viewpoint of the patient. Among these models only the Triandis approach seems to be complimentary to the four stage and may be very useful at the point when we try to develop specific remedial interventions that have been identified within the rubric of the four stage model.

The four stage model was refined to suit patient perspectives, but the stages remained in every way parallel to the physician model in conceptualisation. Inter-analyst agreement for sorting patient statements was 81% for all patients.

DEVELOPING A UNITARY MODEL OF THE CLINICAL MANAGEMENT PROCESS

(i) Combining the Physician and Patient Models

Having established by inductive analysis that the four-stage decision model developed for physicians is also the best fit for the management-related statements extracted from patient interviews, we now have two parallel models which can be combined contemporaneously into a joint model. In this combined model (Figure 1) the physician's assessment of the patient's multiple dysfunctions (personal, situational and biochemical) leads to the choice of an appropriate set of goals with or without negotiation with the patient. The patient usually takes the physician's choice of management plan and implementation tactics, modifies them for his own use on a day-to-day

FIGURE 1 Combining the Physician and Patient Models

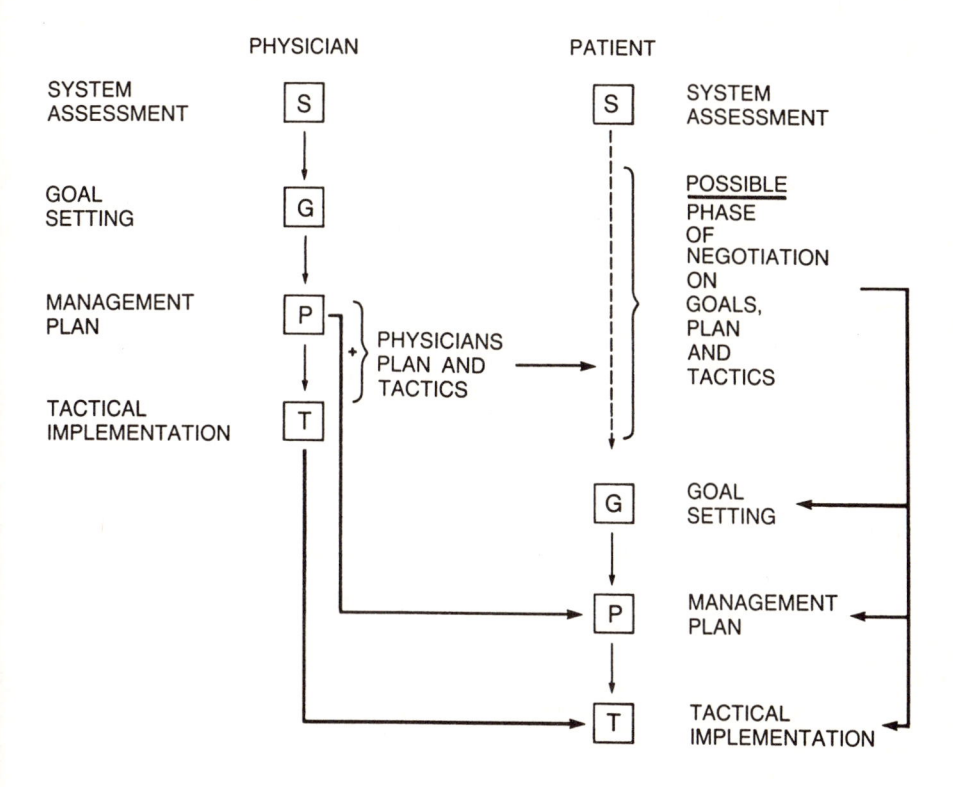

FIGURE 1 (diagram):

PHYSICIAN column:
- SYSTEM ASSESSMENT — S
- GOAL SETTING — G
- MANAGEMENT PLAN — P
- TACTICAL IMPLEMENTATION — T

PATIENT column:
- SYSTEM ASSESSMENT — S
- POSSIBLE PHASE OF NEGOTIATION ON GOALS, PLAN AND TACTICS
- GOAL SETTING — G
- MANAGEMENT PLAN — P
- TACTICAL IMPLEMENTATION — T

Physicians Plan and Tactics → Patient.

---

basis and reports back periodically to the physician on the success or failure of reaching the goals implicit in the management plan. Patients may or may not have a degree of managerial flexibility in modifying diet or medication in the light of feedback from for example, home glucose monitoring.

(ii) Modeling the Disease Process

Engel (1980) has developed, over a period of years, his systems view of illness and disease (Figure 2). Systems are interrelated and are arranged in an interactive hierarchy. The impact of an illness such as diabetes occurs at many different levels. There can be early mild forms and later more complex and irreversible forms of dysfunction. A physician with a strongly biomedical orientation might concentrate most of his attention on the biochemical and lower levels of system organisation (Figure 2) while a psychosocially orientated physician might focus on the upper levels. It can probably be asserted that a broadly based comprehensive assessment of all levels is desirable.

FIGURE 2 **A Multi-level General Systems Model**

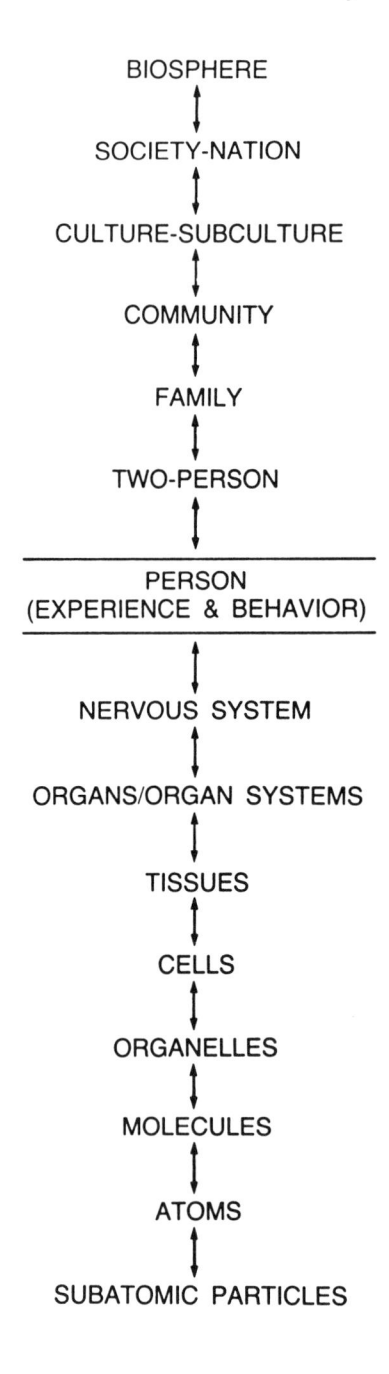

BIOSPHERE
↕
SOCIETY-NATION
↕
CULTURE-SUBCULTURE
↕
COMMUNITY
↕
FAMILY
↕
TWO-PERSON
↕
───────────────────────
PERSON
(EXPERIENCE & BEHAVIOR)
───────────────────────
↕
NERVOUS SYSTEM
↕
ORGANS/ORGAN SYSTEMS
↕
TISSUES
↕
CELLS
↕
ORGANELLES
↕
MOLECULES
↕
ATOMS
↕
SUBATOMIC PARTICLES

The threat of a disease or a pathological process results in a serious dislocation of one or more systems, with resulting dysfunctions. This systems approach is contrasted with the mechanistic biomedical model which focuses on cause/effect relationships in disease, resulting in a continuous search for specific causes and cures for disease. This proved very productive with acute infective diseases, but is of limited value when applied to chronic diseases and their management. The concepts of challenge, adaptation, accommodation and dysfunction are basic to a view of illness based on systems and their management.

There obviously can be conflicts between the physician and the patient as to which dysfunctions are most important. Any attempt to direct the patient in a way that conflicts with the patient's own set of priorities about managing his illness will result in conflict and probably lack of adherence to the proposed management plan. Challenges, events, stimuli, adaptation, accommodation, signals, equilibrium states and functional levels are all the language of modern biology. Diabetologists now talk about one pancreatic cell population, for example, beta cells, "talking to", "adapting" or "accommodation" to the functional state of another cell population such as alpha cells. Investigators talk about glucose challenges to the glucose counter-regulatory system of the pancreas. This systems view of disease can be illustrated by a number of examples.

The onset of dysfunction in diabetes is manifested by signals emanating from the patient at multiple systems levels. For example, hypoglycemia might cause recurrent cognitive dysfunction, producing problems within a marriage or with school work. Other signals of hypoglycemia include sweating, nausea, tachycardia. The patient interprets the signals and if necessary calls in the aid of the physician in making a diagnosis. Both for the physician and the patient there is an "action" threshold for signals above which a significant event or dysfunction is presumed to be happening. The process of managment decision-making is then initiated to identify the diagnosis of system status before deciding how to adjust the management of the problem. In this way, the biological system model can be seen to be interacting with both the physician and patient decision models (Figure 3).

(iii) Combining all Three Processes: physician, patient and disease

The processes of physician and patient decision-making and the metabolic disease process and its resulting dysfunctions are integrated into one general systems model in Figure 3. This views the disease and its management within one unitary multi-level model.

Down the centre of Figure 3 is represented the organism (i.e. the patient) viewed at several different levels. When a significant event occurs in the patient's life, for example, a visit to a relative, a viral syndrome episode or a car accident, this has multiple impacts. It produces a challenge to the current equilibrium state. As the

FIGURE 3 Unitary Multi-level Multi-system Model of Diabetes Management

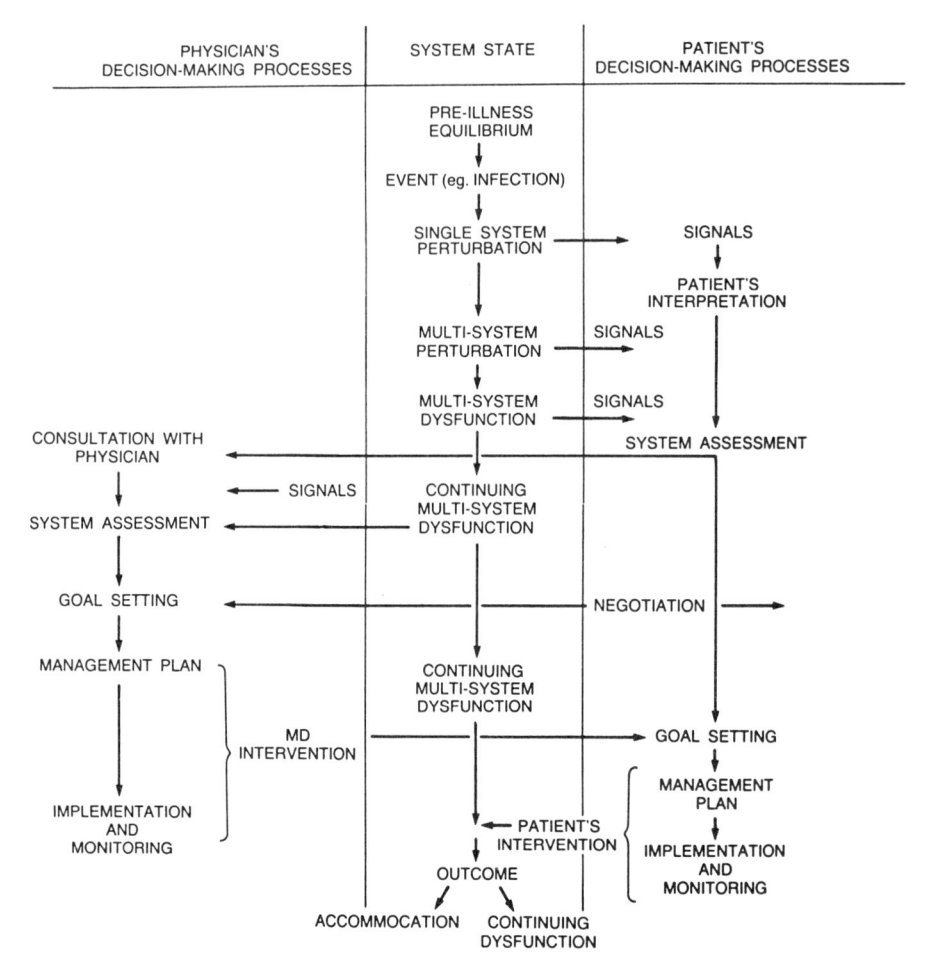

PHYSICIAN'S DECISION-MAKING PROCESSES	SYSTEM STATE	PATIENT'S DECISION-MAKING PROCESSES
	PRE-ILLNESS EQUILIBRIUM ↓	
	EVENT (eg. INFECTION) ↓	
	SINGLE SYSTEM PERTURBATION →	SIGNALS ↓ PATIENT'S INTERPRETATION
	MULTI-SYSTEM PERTURBATION →	SIGNALS
	MULTI-SYSTEM DYSFUNCTION →	SIGNALS
CONSULTATION WITH PHYSICIAN ↓		SYSTEM ASSESSMENT
SYSTEM ASSESSMENT ← SIGNALS ↓	CONTINUING MULTI-SYSTEM DYSFUNCTION	
GOAL SETTING ↓		NEGOTIATION
MANAGEMENT PLAN ⎤ ↓ ⎥ MD INTERVENTION ⎥ ↓ ⎥ IMPLEMENTATION AND MONITORING ⎦	CONTINUING MULTI-SYSTEM DYSFUNCTION ↓ ← PATIENT'S INTERVENTION ↓ OUTCOME ↙ ↘ ACCOMMOCATION CONTINUING DYSFUNCTION	GOAL SETTING ↓ MANAGEMENT PLAN ↓ IMPLEMENTATION AND MONITORING

impacts of the event affect other levels in the system hierarchy there may be a (i) prompt return to equilibrium, (ii) some level of adaptation or (iii) some kind of dysfunction. All this time of perturbation the systems at all levels are emitting signals both to the patient and often to the observant physician. The patient then attempts to make some kind of system assessment (see left hand column of Figure 3). The physician, if he is contacted and asked to intervene, begins the process of arriving at a system assessment in the light of the signals available to him from all levels of the patient. He begins, as in any problem-solving situation, a process of hypothesis testing (or "signal sampling") to develop his overall system assessment (including the available resources and likely obstacles to treatment). He then moves through the process of "goal setting" taking account of the impact of the illness at all levels of the patient's functioning to arrive at a management plan and appropriate tactics for its implementation and monitoring (left hand column, Figure 3).

At this stage, the patient is in a kind of "stall" between making his/her own system assessment and awaiting the outcome of the analysis of the problem by the physician. They usually delay initiating their own process of goal setting until they are presented with an assessment and management plan/implementation package by the physician. A "negotiation" process may have gone on between physician and patient to obtain concensus on goals (although our video data suggest this is rare). Patients usually proceed with the physician's plan and develop their own evaluation of it over a period of weeks or months. They may then modify all or part of it to suit their own goals and lifestyle. Such plans then become the intervention by the patient in their own illness. This action/intervention leads to a process of accommodation or adaptation to the illness resulting in an acceptable equilibrium/adaptation outcome state at all significant levels.

A general systems model such as this allows us to accommodate all three critical elements in one model incorporating the decision-making systems of patients, physicians and the overall systems perspective of the patient and his/her illness.

(iv) Illustrative Case Study and Analysis Case Study

The concepts of challenge, adaptation, accommodation and dysfunction are obviously critical to this systems view of illness. This systems view of disease and illness and the role of the physician and patient in managing it has been used to analyse a case study.

A patient in her middle fifties (one of our interview sample) was very poorly controlled and had chronic problems with weight control and leg pain (diabetic neuropathy). The patient has a 28-year-old son who is a drug addict to whom she is very over-protective. She was unable to come to grips with her dietary restrictions and was put on insulin. She continues to be in poor metabolic control and to gain weight. The amount of insulin necessary to keep her blood sugar under control continues to increase. The physician has tried many manoeuvres, including education, psychotherapy, motivational talks and books, and was completely frustrated in his attempt to motivate the patient to give up her dependent relationship with her son and to face up to controlling her diabetes.

This is a good example of multi-system dysfunction. As far as the patient is concerned, a normal adult relationship between herself and her son is unacceptable. This may be because of her own past history or that of her son. This infant-mother relationship is dysfunctional for both and results in her developing a chronic tension state with a diversion of emotional and intellectual resources away from control of her type II diabetes. Her physician is aware of this and correctly decided that simply dealing with the problem at the metabolic level was not going to solve the problem of ineffective control.

Here we have an example of conflict between the physician's notion of acceptable goals and system states and those of his patient. The patient is quite willing to settle for dysfunction at one level (namely the neurotic relationship with her son) at the expense of equilibrium at other more metabolic levels. She is also quite willing to accept the long-term consequences of chronic poor control, but is quite unwilling to accept the short-term emotional consequences of giving up a dysfunctional relationship with her son. Figure 4 illustrates the different systems involved in her ongoing illness, including an estimate of the relative and often conflicting priorities of physicians and patients about problems. For example, at the two-person system level (dyad) she has difficulty with her physician. She also has person level difficulties with appetite and weight control and is poorly informed about diabetes. At a tissue level she has several problems with her glucose regulatory system. At an organ level she also has concomitant biomedical disturbances associated with her non-insulin dependent diabetes, e.g. neuropathy. To bring the family system (which is in chronic dysequilibrium) into a more stable state, would involve her giving up her current role as a mother. As far as the patient (in her interview) is concerned, if she is not a mother she is a "non-entity". She, therefore, is not prepared to relinquish her motherhood role with her son. Her physician has recognised this and feels that until she changes her relationship with her son, she will be unable to devote the energy necessary to bring her appetite and weight under control. This must occur to allow her to cut back on the high level of inslin that she is taking because of her chronic lack of control.

DEFINITION OF CLINICAL JUDGMENT IN MANAGEMENT DECISION-MAKING

To make a clinical judgment using our unitary systems model is then seen as a process of assessing accurately and appropriately the range of dysfunctions to arrive at an overall system assessment. This forms the basis for integrating all elements and levels of the patient's illness to allow the selection of appropriate goals from which the management plan will follow. Such a view of clinical judgement as "integration" is particularly compatible with the description by Cluff (1978), "To state the biochemical, physiological, molecular, subcellular and other important facts about a disease, however, is not difficult. To analyse, co-ordinate, integrate and orchestrate this knowledge into patient management is difficult. Physicians are very naturally reticent on such matters, slow to commit their thoughts to paper and very suspicious of any attempt to tabulate their methods of reasoning. Yet these processes are the ones essential for personal care and must be then demonstrated to those learning to become physicians".

SYSTEM DYSFUNCTIONS

	DIABETES RELATED	M.D.	PAT.	OTHERS	M.D.	PAT.
FAMILY				SON'S HEROIN ADDICTION	1	5
				FAMILY DYSFUNCTION	3	5
TWO PERSON				DOCTOR/PATIENT CONFLICT	1	4
PERSON	APPETITE/WT. CONTROL	5	3	LOW SELF-ESTEEM	4	5
	DIETARY COMPLIANCE	5	3			
	EDUCATION RE: DIABETES	1	1			
SYSTEMS	IATROGENIC INSULIN ADMINISTRATION	4	1			
ORGAN	NEUROPATHY (LEG PAIN)	4	4			
TISSUE	RECEPTOR DEFICIT	1	1			
	CIRCULATING INSULIN ANTAGONISTS	1	1			
	LATE BETA CELL FAILURE	1	1			
CELL	INTRACELLULAR DEFICIT IN GLUCOSE METABOLISM	1	1			
	DECREASE IN NUMBER OF INSULIN RECEPTORS (IN LIVER, FAT, MUSCLE CELLS)	1	1			

RELATIVE IMPORTANCE RELATIVE IMPORTANCE
5 = VERY IMPORTANT   1 = LITTLE IMPORTANCE

Figure 4 Summary of multi-level dysfunction in illustrative case with estimates (from analysis of interview transcripts in the study) of relative importance of dysfunctions to patient and physician

SALIENT FEATURES OF THE MANAGEMENT MODEL

1. A greatly broadened system-orientated view of diagnosis and prognosis.
2. A primacy of goal setting and value hierarchies.
3. The physician's decision-making role emphasises "integration" of multiple goals into a co-ordinated plan.
4. A clear distinction between the management intervention and the choice of tactics for its implementation and monitoring.
5. A descriptive/transactional view of physician/patient communication and negotiation of goals which avoids favouring any specific style or approach by the physician.
6. A descriptive approach which combines both process and descriptive perspectives on the clinical decision-making.

ANALYSIS OF VIDEO RECORDING OF ROUTINE CLINIC VISITS

(i) Methods

We made video recordings of clinic visits on a random sample of eight out of the twenty-four physician/patient pairs. These video recordings were reviewed by both physician and patient. Stimulated recalls were conducted on these clinic visit videotapes on the same day in the physician's office and later the same day in the patient's home. These videotapes and their stimulated recall audiotapes have been of considerable value in validating some of our findings and demonstrating the application of the four-stage management model in practice.

In the stimulated recall method, an event (such as a clinic visit) is videotaped and the participant reviews the videotape very soon afterwards. The videotaped replay of the event stimulates visit recall of covert thoughts, emotions and other responses as they occurred moment-by-moment during the original event. With the prompting of a trained "inquirer", these responses are expressed and captured on audiotape. The combination of the videotaped encounter and simultaneous interpretation of events by participants provides an unusually rich database. These data can suggest the factors which influence the subject's decision-making under "real world" conditions. This method is now well established as a means of investigating cognitive, emotional and attitudinal dynamics which underlie behaviour.

These videotapes and stimulated recalls were completed at the time of the original interviews before any content analysis was done. They preceded the development of the management model by 18 months. We decided to use the videotape data to attempt to validate our four-stage model for the physician.

(ii) Results of Qualitative Analysis of Video and Recall Tapes

As with the original interviews, virtually all verbal transactions of the visit could be reliably categorised within the rubric of the model, with the exception of social interchanges, discussions about matters unrelated to diabetes and transactions which involve the actual delivery of interventions to the patient.

With well controlled, "easy to manage" patients, physicians usually proceeded through the familiar sequence of history, physical exam, laboratory studies and recommendations with obvious attention to the issues of assessment, plans and tactics. References to goal setting were rarely found on the videotaped encounters, but were frequently discussed by physicians as justifications for their actions during the stimulated recall sessions. Stimulated recall sessions in the treatment of such well controlled patients confirmed and, to some extent, extended our understanding of the model's application in practice, but provided no fundamentally new insights.

With problematic patients, however, physicians appeared to move in unpredictable order from one stage of our model to another and from one content area to another. The stimulated recall sessions with physicians demonstrated, however, that such digressions were anything but haphazard. Instead, we saw evidence that all physicians worked from a coherent set of assumptions, goals, plans and tactics which comported with our model, but at the same time they were alert to new leads that might result in progress related to any stage. Thus, it appears that the four-stage model provides a template for orderly consideration of a routine case and when challenged by a significant management problem, that physicians can and do move with great flexibility from stage to stage within this framework.

(iii) Conclusions

As a heuristic device the four-stage model provided a framework for making the following observations about management decision-making.
1. The importance of re-establishing a fresh assessment in the earliest moments of each visit appears paramount. One physician in the stimulated recall session described himself as "struggling like fury to get on top of (the case)" as he casually paged through the chart and engaged the patient in small talk.
2. The goals of physicians were frequently pursued without attempts to understand whether the goals of the patient were compatible. Physicians routinely responded to the question "What do you think the patient wanted?" with "I don't know".
3. Physicians experienced the greatest frustration when their assessments and goals did not suggest any reasonable plan to them. Under such circumstances, several physician responses have been observed including
    a) casting about for some point of intervention even without a plan,
    b) intervening strongly to deliberately perturb the status quo and create a new situation for which a plan might be forthcoming,
    c) redefining the problem, thereby recasting the goals and devising a dramatically different plan and
    d) remaining frustrated and often instilling guilt into the patient.
4. Physicians may expend considerable energy working out plans and devising ingenious implementation tactics while recognising that they are not "getting through to the patient". Stimulated recall sessions and other interviews with patients have revealed that the patient's assessment and/or goals in such cases can be fundamentally incompatible with the assessments and goals of the physician to which the physician's plans and implementation tactics are addressed.

APPLICATION OF THE MANAGEMENT MODEL

The most useful and immediate application of the management decision model is that we have been able to identify important stages in the development of a management policy. The system assessment stage of the management process is an elaboration of the diagnosis and problem-solving aspects of clinical decision-making which have been so extensively explored (reviewed in detail by Elstein et al., 1978). However, there is no pre-existing theoretical basis for the goal setting stage of clinical management, which we have identified, other than the decision analytic concept of "subjective expected utility".

Reviewing the literature, we found almost no systematic analysis of the topic of goal setting in chronic disease management in either the health services or the clinical care literature, yet 39% of all the statements by physicians fell into this category indicating that physicians regard it as being of considerable clinical importance. Stages 3 and 4 (the management plan and tactical implementation) were judged to be as a consequence of a chosen set of assessments and goals and will be studied in detail later. Development of instruments to measure both physician and patient goal setting is well advanced and will be reported elsewhere (Taylor et al., to be published).

FUTURE USES OF THE MODEL

Given that we have derived a four-stage management decision model inductively from both patient and physician interview data with high interjudge reliability, we are faced with the problem of deciding how to validate such a model. The model clearly has attractive heuristic value in the sense that it allows the process of management to be studied within quite distinct although highly interrelated stages with different categories of cognitive data. The two models can be combined with a systems description of diabetes into a general dynamic systems model of clinical management as we have shown. We hope to continue to use the model as a way of looking at the management process in diabetes care, but also to develop measures of beliefs and preferences of physicians and patients at different stages of the process.

Currently we are actively developing profile generating measures for both physicians and patients for both system assessment and the goal setting stages of the process (Figure 5). They will allow us to measure how compatible physicians and patients are at these important stages of management and will allow us to shift attention from a normative to a descriptive approach to doctor/patient interaction. Much of the literature on doctor/patient communication and interaction assumes that there is a specific highly desirable way in which the physician should relate to the patient. The style of relationship advocated is usually characterised as being open to negotiation, tolerant, non-paternalistic and non-authoritarian.

Figure 5 **Four-stage Model and Profile Generating Instruments**

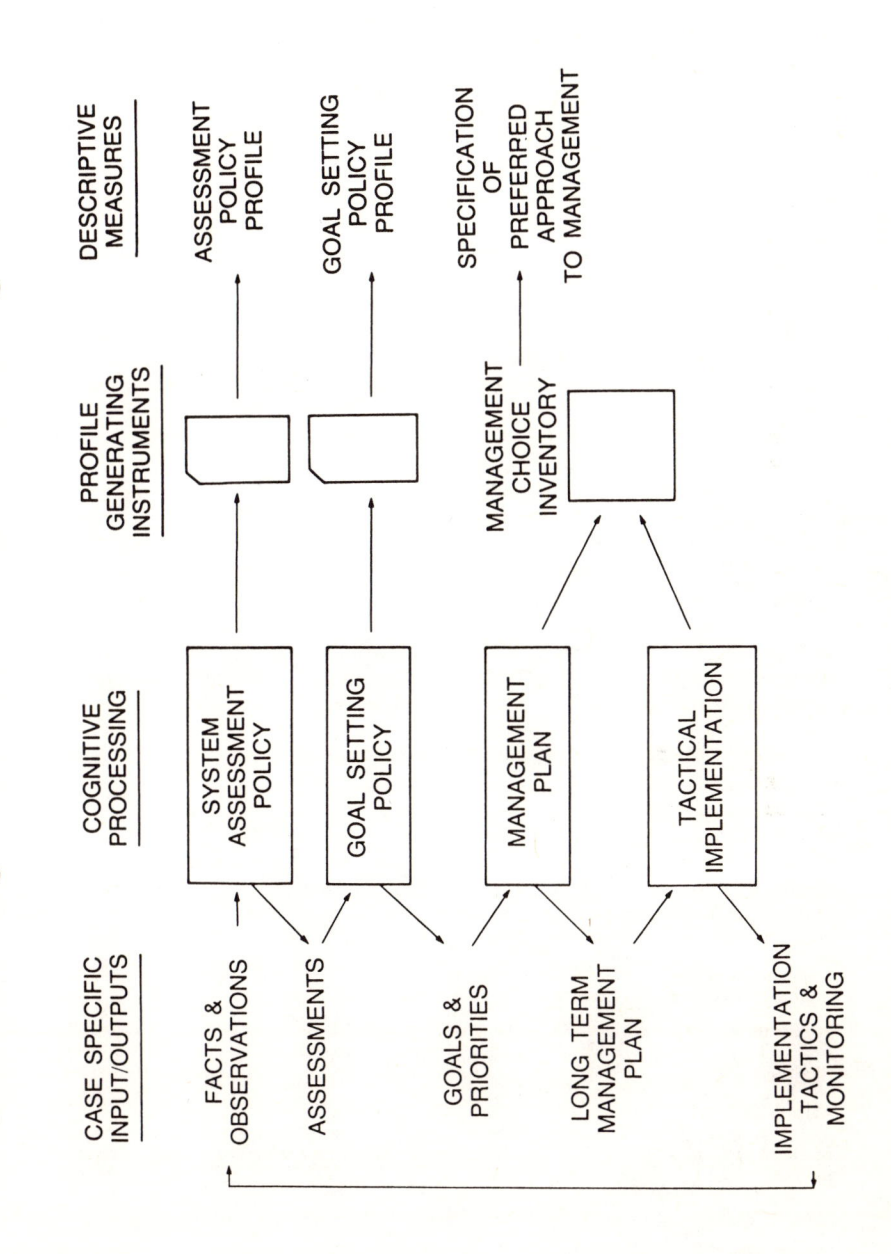

Our approach will be to describe as accurately and as objectively as possible (using our profile generating measures, Figure 5) effective styles of doctor/patient relationship. We hypothesise that patients with comparable severity of disease will do better when their goals and expectations are compatible with those of their physician rather than incompatible. We plan to test these hypotheses in future studies. We see such studies as a method of indirectly validating our model's assumptions about the management process.

REFERENCES

Barrows, H.S., and Abrahamson, S., (1964). The programmed patient. Journal of Medical Education, 39: 802-805.

Barrows, H.S., and Bennett, K., (1972). The diagnostic (problem-solving) skill of the neurologist: experimental studies and their implications for neurological training. Archives of Neurology, 26: 270-277.

Beach, L.R. (1982). Decision-making: diagnosis, action selection and implementation. Choice Models for Buyer Behaviour. Research in Marketing, Supplement No. 1, 185-200.

Cluff, L.E. (1978). The integrative function of the physicians in making medical decisions. The Pharos, 2-4: (October) 1978.

Einhorn, H.J., Kleinmuntz, D.H., and Kleinmuntz, B. (1979). Linear regression and process-tractin models of judgement. Psychological Review, 86: 465-485.

Einhorn, H.J., and Hogarth, R.M. (1981). Behavioural decision theory: processes of judgement and choice. Annual Review of Psychology, 32: 53-88, 1981.

Elstein, A.S., Shulman, L.S., and Sprafka, S.A. (1978). Medical Problem-Solving: An Analysis of Clinical Reasoning. Cambridge, MA: Harvard University Press.

Engel, G.L. (1980). The clinical application of the biopsychosocial model. American Journal of Psychiatry, 137: 535.

Kirkwood, C.R., Clure, H.R., Brodsky, R. et. al., (1982). The diagnostic content of family practices. Journal of Family Practice, 15: 485-492.

Mintzberg, H., (1973). The Nature of Managerial Work. London: Harper and Row.

15
The Probabilistic Paradigm as the Basic Science of the Practice of Family Medicine

Richard I. Feinbloom

I would like to propose in my paper a framework for clinical practice which is grounded in the fundamental principles of twentieth century science. From this framework we can derive a coherent, unified, integrated, consistent approach to patient care, a science of practice. We can prune, recontextualise and reorganise the patchwork quilt of concepts and practices such as compliance, placebo effect, iatrogenesis and patients' rights which have proliferated in recent years in an effort to clarify problematic issues. In this analysis I will examine aspects of our contemporary conventional wisdom, expose some of its contradictions and produce a blueprint which is elegant in its simplicity, sharp in its rigour and immediately applicable. To be specific, I want to propose that we apply the science of our time to the clinical setting, a science which stems ultimately from work in theoretical physics and can be described as the probabilistic paradigm, as distinguished from its predecessor, the mechanistic paradigm.

In this presentation I want to acknowledge the contributions of Harold Bursztajn, Robert Hamm, and Archie Brodsky with whom I have worked on these ideas and their application over the past ten years. Bursztajn and Hamm, (1979); Bursztajn et al, (1981) What follows is based on this collaboration.

At the turn of this century, physicists found themselves in the quandary of being unable to predict the behavior of subatomic particles with the earlier Newtonian rules. In the resulting paradigm shift, a science of absolute certainty gave way to one of probability. Unicausality yielded to multicausality. Chance and cause became complementary instead of being mutually exclusive. The observer no longer stood outside of the experiment but became part of it. Subjective factors became as legitimate a concern for science as objective factors. The previous dichotomy between objectivity and subjectivity disappeared.

This paradigm shift in the physical sciences has strongly influenced medical practice. We have, for example, come to view the search for a single cause ("magic bullet") for a given effect as simplistic. We have abandoned the view of the doctor-scientist as a detached observer and now recognise that the physician exerts a strong placebo effect which, as Michael Balint has pointed out, may be the most powerful drug of all. We now make it a point to pay much more attention to the patient's feelings and not simply to objective data such as electrocardiogram and serum electrolytes. And we have incorporated into practice notions such as compliance, patients' rights, informed consent, patient advocacy and decision analysis. All of these important developments can be viewed as evidence of a shift from a mechanistic to a probabilistic model.

However, in medicine this shift is incomplete. We are still strongly gripped by our mechanistic inheritance. The very concepts and practices which I advanced to demonstrate the shift from mechanistic to probabilistic can, when viewed in a slightly different light, be seen to represent transitional forms between the two paradigms with strong persisting elements of mechanistic thinking. For example, the concept of compliance recognises that not all prescriptions are filled or are taken as prescribed, a disturbing fact for the mechanistic mind which finds such uncertainty intolerable. On the other hand, if the principles of compliance are followed, the errant patient's behaviour becomes predictable and controllable. Certainty is restored. Viewed from the perspective of the probabilistic paradigm, concepts such as compliance can be seen as last ditch attempts to shore up a crumbling mechanistic approach, analogous to the efforts of physicists in the early 1900s to bend Newtonian mechanics to explain the motion of subatomic particles.

In our book, "Medical Choices, Medical Chances", (Bursztajn et al., 1981) we report our experience with a practice brought into alignment with the criteria of the probabilistic paradigm. Each of the major criteria of this paradigm, which in our analysis are three in number (and have their counterparts in the mechanistic paradigm) have specific implications for practice.

The first criterion of the probabilistic paradigm acknowledges uncertainty at the core of the universe. Although we can never know for sure, we need not despair. We are capable of making decisions under conditions of uncertainty by converting uncertainty to probability. In fact we do so all of the time. Only some of the time, however, is this decision-making made explicitly. For example, we are used to weather forecasts of a "ninety percent chance of rain" upon which we base a decision of what to do or wear.

The formal method of deciding under conditions of uncertainty is decision analysis. Decision analysis is, at least today, of little use in most clinical settings where precise probabilities of risks and benefits are not available, formal clarification of values takes too long, and decision trees exist only for a handful of problems.

While in no way discouraging the further application of decision analysis, we suggest that diagnostic and therapeutic choices are better seen as acts of gambling. The linguistic metaphor of gambling can accurately describe medical decision-making and has the advantage of high public recognition. People know about betting and odds and can easily make the jump from the race track to the consultation suite. Furthermore, gambling expresses very well the act of subjective probability assessment which describes how we make decisions in our everyday lives.

The probabilistic physician and patient, in short, are unabashed gamblers. They gamble above the table, in a fully conscious state, and recognise the influence of various gambling errors such as post mortem hindsight and the "gambler's fallacy". The smart gambler also takes into account recent findings in cognitive psychology which identify irrational factors affecting preferences such as the impact on choices of how problems are formulated or "framed". For example, stating identical outcomes in terms of the chance of survival as opposed to the chance of death has been demonstrated to alter the choices people make between alternative therapies (McNeil et al, 1982).

The gambling metaphor can be applied readily to the most common problems, such as the care of a sore throat. The doctor formulates the various options with costs and benefits, such as neither culture nor treat with antibiotics; culture and treat, and revise treatment according to the culture report; treat without culturing; culture and treat only if the culture is positive. Risks and benefits include penicillin allergy, financial expense, the discomfort of a culture, predictive value of a culture, the prevention of sequlae and feeling better quicker. Which gamble to make depends also on the patient's values. A person with a major board meeting or opera recital scheduled for the next day may be willing to accept the risk of a penicillin reaction for the possible benefit of feeling even slightly improved. In this way a choice is negotiated.

Sharing uncertainty with patients spells the end of the physician as manager and the beginning of the physician as broker of choice. It is also the end of compliance and informed consent. What meaning do such concepts have under conditions of informed choice? Such is the impact of a paradigm shift.

The second criterion of the probabilistic paradigm is drawn from Heisenberg's famous principle of uncertainty, which explains that the velocity of an electron changes when its position is observed and vice versa. Position and velocity cannot be predicted simultaneously. Gone forever is the validity of the belief in an objective world uninfluenced by observation.

Experienced clinicians know the therapeutic effect of listening, i.e. observing. Simply listening can produce a cure. The experienced clinician is also aware of his own personal placebo effect, i.e. the mere presence of the doctor can be therapeutic.

According to the second criterion, the observer effect is intrinsic to observation. It is unavoidable. The question is not whether one has an impact through observation but whether one will be responsible and accountable for it, whether the observer effect will be consciously considered and used for the benefit of the patient.

Doctors for many years have sought the ideal of objectivity, as though they should know a patient independently of their own feelings and beliefs. Under the second criterion, physicians can unburden themselves of this illusion. They are encouraged to be themselves and to be in touch with their feelings and how these affect the patient. The relationship between doctor and patient can be brought into the limelight for scrutiny. The critical issue of trust, for example, can be freely discussed instead of being taboo. Just as it is necessary for the doctor to admit that he is only 95% confident that a suggested diagnosis is accurate, he can take the initiative in raising the question of a second opinion and can check on the patient's satisfaction with the consultation process. In other words, it is all right and even at times necessary to talk about the relationship as a factor in the decision-making process. Furthermore, the reduction of uncertainty in the relationship frees both doctor and patient to apply their energies to coping with the real clinical uncertainty which faces them both.

Being accountable for the impact that he has on the patient and using it for the patient's best interests, the physician now functions consistently with the spirit of modern science. The observer effect, not stated in so many words, has passed over the years in the guise of the art of medicine, outside of science. Under the probabilistic paradigm it is included in the science of practice.

The transformational impact of the paradigm shift on conventional thinking is also apparent with criterion two. For example, we traditionally make a distinction between diagnostic and treatment measures. Under the probabilistic paradigm, the distinction between diagnosis and treatment diappears. To diagnose is to treat and to treat is to diagnose. We are familiar with the therapeutic trial which makes a diagnosis and with the therapeutic impact of simply knowing a diagnosis. Visualisation of the bile ducts, i.e. observation, and bypassing obstructions within them, i.e. treatment, are part and parcel of the same technical manoeuvre. We also are now keenly aware of the fact that there is no free lunch with diagnostic measures. They have risks and benefits just as does therapy. Only a model of science which sees the observer as outside of the experiment would lead one to think otherwise.

The third of the closely related criteria of the probabilistic paradigm is that subjective and objective reality are seen to be on a continuum rather than viewed as dichotomous. Elements of objectivity and subjectivity are present in all knowledge. The electrocardiogram requires interpretation which is rarely as certain as one may think. Paying attention to the anxiety level of the myocardial infarction victim can be as critical in determining his fate as the proper interpretation of his electrocardiogram. No longer need we defer to the art of medicine to justify paying attention to subjective factors. Under the probabilistic paradigm, such a concern finds support from the "hardest" branch of science.

To summarise, medical practice under the probabilistic paradigm rigorously applied would look different in many ways from medical practice today. Drawing the full implications of the paradigm shift would have a profound effect on the way in which patients and doctors relate. Uncertainty would be acknowledged as the starting place for medical decision-making rather than as an intolerable psychological state to be avoided at all costs. Medical decisions would be viewed as gambles. Doctor and patient would gamble together in the interest of the patient in a spirit of fully informed choice that acknowledges the benefits and risks of fully displayed options. Clarification of values would be seen as important as the correct assignment of probabilities for benefits and risks. Gambling would be done consciously taking advantage of research into the psychology of making decisions under conditions of uncertainty. The observer effect would be acknowledged and would be taken into account in the clinical setting. Subjective considerations would be given equal weight with objective measures. The art of medicine would be subsumed under the new science of practice.

The risks and benefits of making this leap into twentieth century science are many and cannot be discussed here. Suffice it to say that as clinicians who profess being scientific in their practice, we should, at the very least, pay attention to what science is today. As family physicians we are presented with the opportunity to invigorate our discipline with a new scientific rigour which could become our calling card.

REFERENCES

Bursztajn, H. and Hamm, R. M. (1979) Two Views of Science. Yale Journal of Biology and Science, 52, pp 483-486.

Bursztajn, H.., Feinbloom, R., Hamm, R. and Brodsky, A. (1981). Medical Choices, Medical Chances. How Patients, Families and Physicians can cope with Uncertainty. Delacorte Press/Seymour Lawrence, New York.

McNeil, B.J., Pauker, S.G., Sox, H.C., and Tversky, A. (1982). On the elicitation of preferences for alternative therapies. New Engand Journal of Medicine; 306: 1259-1262.

16
Discussion of the Papers by Taylor and Feinbloom

B.J. Essex

Professor Taylor's paper stimulated a discussion that centred around the question of applicability of this model to other health problems and other users including general practitioners. The same questions relate to the claims made for the probabilistic paradigm described by Feinbloom. Taylor stressed that the value of a model can be measured by the extent to which it helps us to understand complex multifactorial phenomena. Such ill-defined areas pervade the field of primary care and impinge upon many decisions made by doctor and patient alike. If the model has much explanatory power then it may be of use in constructing an agenda for shared decision-making between doctor and patient. However, what became clear in the discussions was the need to measure how far such models did what we thought they ought to do? We need to know where their strengths and weaknesses lie. We also need to study the decisions and problems which fall outside these models, and the frequency with which this occurs. Even when these questions have been answered, more research will have to be done to discover how to use them in the most effective and acceptable way.

Feinbloom's paper presented a probabilistic approach to shared decision-making between doctor and patient. This opened up a discussion on how to explain risks of alternative management options to patients in a way that facilitates informed consent. It was pointed out that information overload can be counter-productive, and that the legal system has a big impact on the ways in which information is selected and presented to patients. The ways in which the doctor presents risks and options to the patient is affected by the value judgments of both and efforts have been made to develop booklet question and answer formats that try to reduce the influence of these important factors. However, these have only very limited application at present. Some of the participants felt that it was important to recognise that some patients will not want to discuss risks and that it is not always appropriate to do so. Occasionally the patient will abrogate this responsibility for making decisions to the doctor. One interesting area of further research is to discover if risk explanation and shared decision-making in planning management increases compliance or not. It was felt that the value of the probabilities approach presented here lies in highlighting the need for more information about the risks and benefits of alternative strategies.

17
The Surface Anatomy of Primary Health Care — Does Consultation Analysis Contribute?

Nigel C.H. Stott

The consultation is often viewed as the hub of Primary Health Care (P.H.C.) around which all other activities revolve and upon which the smooth operation of teamwork depends. The P.H.C. physician has no monopoly over the consultation as nurses, health visitors, assistants, counsellors, therapists, etc. all 'consult' in their various roles. However, physicians have played a major part in developing our understanding of consulting events and it is physicians who have most exposed themselves to the tape-recorder, the observer and the video-camera in a systematic and objective assessment of their interactions with patients. Those who have opened their professional doors in this way need special recognition because allowing yourself to be viewed during clinical encounters brings ruthless scientific scrutiny into a delicate area of dual human behaviour. You may be an authoritarian dogmatic clinician or a sensitive negotiating physician, your style could be 'open' or 'closed', conventional or unconventional. Nevertheless, when you allow others to look and measure and comment, you run certain risks.

Many good and experienced clinicians feel that the process of consultation analysis will gradually lead to consensus views on desirable and less desirable behaviour and this could turn to demands to censor those who are least like the norms established by an intellectual minority (shades of '1984'?). To me the greatest threat is not the research which helps us understand and describe consulting events, but those quasi-academic individuals who seize on every fragment of innovation which can be fitted into their preconceived ideas. Preliminary research results then become combined in 'official' reports and documents and the process of scientific advance becomes pushed, hurried and easily misconstrued. I believe that we stand at this very corner in consultation analysis - an exciting scientific moment for those with the integrity to go on building a sound wall of understanding, and yet a dangerous moment because many ambitious people are beginning to snatch at fragments of evidence to build a new shrine to themselves or their institutions without due humility and without rigorous scientific proof for the validity of their generalisations.

Consultation Analysis - Two Paths

The consultation can be viewed in two broadly different ways: by looking inward in depth or by looking outward in breadth. Both are perfectly valid ways of looking at the consultation but each can result in conclusions with differing priorities. In this paper, I will attempt to provide a view of the two approaches by drawing on research data generated largely in the Department of General Practice at the Welsh National School of Medicine.

Consultation as Communication (or Looking Inwards in Depth)

Video-tape and audio-tape recordings have been used in many ways to analyse the doctor-patient interaction as an exercise in communication, and in Wales we have developed rating scales which can be used by independent raters to assess various components of the consultation. Table 1 summarises the seventeen items which are used on a four-point scale to produce scores from 0-3 with a theoretical

Table 1   General practice interview rating scale

$A : B : C : D$

1 Beginning of interview poor	——:——:——:——	Beginning positive and smooth
2 Seating arrangement open	——:——:——:——	Seating arrangement closed
3 Body posture bad	——:——:——:——	Body posture good
4 Appropriate use of eye contact	——:——:——:——	No eye contact or excessive use of eye contact
5 Frequent use of jargon	——:——:——:——	Absence of jargon
6 Frequently interrupted patient	——:——:——:——	Did not interrupt patient
7 Did not use facilitation	——:——:——:——	Frequent use of facilitation
8 Encouraged patient to keep to relevant matter	——:——:——:——	Not able to keep patient to relevant matter
9 Good clarification	——:——:——:——	Lack of clarification
10 Did not cover psychosocial areas	——:——:——:——	Covered psychosocial areas
11 Avoided personal issues	——:——:——:——	Did not avoid personal issues
12 No empathic statements	——:——:——:——	Frequent use of empathic statements
13 Picked up leads	——:——:——:——	Failed to pick up leads
14 Time spent in silence inappropriate	——:——:——:——	Appropriate use of silence
15 Good question style	——:——:——:——	Inappropriate question style
16 Warm	——:——:——:——	Cold
17 Ending of interview smooth and definite	——:——:——:——	Ending of interview abrupt or imprecise

maximum of 51 points. This was pioneered by Professor John Verby from Minnesota in collaboration with Professor Harvard Davis and many others in our department in Wales, and a full account of the validation and reliability testing procedures are available elsewhere (Verby, Davis and Holden, 1979). For the purpose of this report, I shall describe the results of two experiments on:

(a) experienced general practitioners

(b) less experienced general practitioners (Verby, Davis and Holden, 1980).

In the first experiment, seventeen experienced general practitioners participated in an experiment to assess the impact of information feedback. Each had a series of consultations recorded in their own practices at intervals of between three and five months. Five of the doctors formed an experimental group which met weekly to view and discuss one another's recordings, while the other twelve doctors formed a control group who did not see their recordings during the study period. One hundred and forty-six complete consultations were recorded and rated from the two groups. The overall results are illustrated in Figure 1 and show that the experimental group achieved a statistically significant change in their mean scores. Most of this change was attributable to variables 7 (facilitation), 9

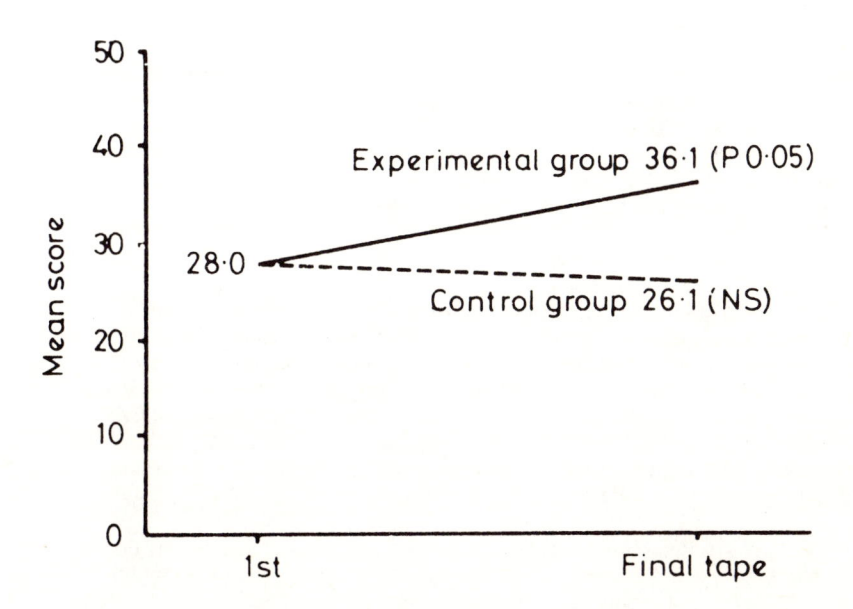

Figure 1 Mean scores of experimental and control groups showing movements from first to final videotapes

(clarification), 13 (ability to pick up verbal and non-verbal leads), 15 (question style), 16 (warmth) and 17 (ending the interview), but non-significant trends in the expected directions were present for most of the other variables.

I conclude from this study that experienced general practitioners are capable of modifying some of their consulting techniques in the face of peer review of recordings. We cannot conclude that this is necessarily beneficial for patient care, although it seems likely that the outcome would be good because conventional wisdom decrees that the change was in a desirable direction. The higher scores were, however, most likely in the longest consultations.

The second study was designed to test the hypothesis that interviewing skills and techniques of young doctors undergoing vocational training for general practice can be improved by specific teaching based on video-tape records of their consultations in the training practices. Nine registrars who formed the experimental group each had six 30-minute consultation sessions recorded at three week intervals. After each session, the tape was viewed and discussed with an experienced teacher (Professor Verby) on a one to one basis. In addition, reading matter was recommended which dealt with interviewing skills. The control group of eight registrars each had two 30-minute recordings at the beginning and end of the study period. No viewing was arranged, and the two groups were similar in age and experience.

One hundred and sixty-five records were rated from the seventeen registrars in this survey, each tape having between two and five consultations on it. Somewhat heterogeneous results emerged from the project as some registrars in both groups improved and others did less well, indicating that unexpected variables were operating to confound the results. The most useful analysis is shown in Figure 2, where a non-significant drift in both groups in the first six-months registrarship is compared with divergent results in the second six-months in both. These differences did not quite reach statistical significance on the mean scores, but an overall decline in the performance of the control groups was a source of concern. An item analysis revealed that the important variables for change in the experimental group were similar to those of the experienced doctors in the first study, but interpretation of these results has to be very cautious in the face of results which were not fully consistent with original hypotheses. It appears that video-consultation feed-back is most productive in the more experienced young doctors but, unlike their older colleagues, there is less relationship between time taken and performance as judged on these scales.

The two studies illustrate how an interview rating scale can be used to measure a number of pre-selected variables, many of which are gradually being incorporated into consensus views of what constitutes good interviewing. Our results also illustrate that great caution has to be exercised in using these data, because the outcome was not altogether consistent with the original hypotheses and the numbers

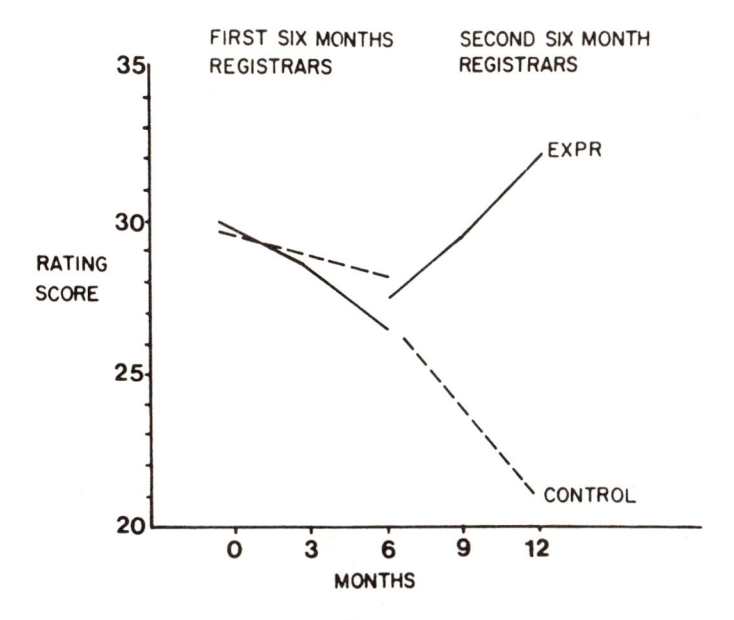

Figure 2 A comparison of the mean scores of the registrars during their training

involved are necessarily small. One of the difficulties with in-depth studies is that the sample size has to be limited and hence the conclusions also have to be cautious until the work has been reproduced in several different population groups. I am sad to report that our work is often quoted by others as evidence for the improvement general practitioners show when given opportunity for self-observation of video-taped consultations. This is true only insofar as it applies to the seventeen criteria on the Cardiff rating scale when applied to more experienced registrars or principals. The important factor of time taken for each consultation and its relationship to rated performance is largely neglected by most of those who have quoted our work, yet this was one of the most important conclusions in the study of experienced principals. The deterioration in measured performance of the control group of registrars was the most startling finding in the second study, yet this too has received scant attention from commentators, perhaps because it fitted least well into preconceived ideas about the impact of vocational training. I make these points here, not because our results are inviolate, but because it is too easy for each of us to pick what is attractive and convenient from the work of others and then to neglect or misconstrue actual results and conclusions.

Decision-making in General Practice

The Technique of Audio-Visual Review

The technique of audio-visual consultation review became more and more important as the Welsh research group reviewed hundreds of video-taped consultations. They grew to recognise that certain ground rules were important (Davis et al. 1980):

(a) That newcomers to the technique must be encouraged to view their tapes alone before being exposed to the comments from a peer group.

(b) That any peer group leader must have had his own consultations recorded and reviewed by others to sensitize him to risks and benefits of video analysis.

(c) That any video-taped consultation is such a brief snapshot of a continuing relationship between doctor and patient that a group must always concentrate on what is present on a tape and refuse to be drawn into debates on what is absent or perceived to be absent.

(d) That the doctor whose tape is being viewed must always initiate peer group discussion.

(e) That stable groups and ad-hoc groups have different needs and dynamics - a point for leaders to study and apply (see Davis et al., 1980, for fuller description).

Each of these ground rules may seem trite to those who have become desensitized to the stress of having a consultation viewed by peers.....but our experience is that they are as valid now as they were in the early days of our work and it is interesting that an Oxford research group have come to very similar conclusions (Pendleton et al., 1983).

Side Effects of Video-Analysis

Most research workers and teachers find that neither doctors nor patients develop adverse feelings about video-analysis of consultations, once they have participated themselves. Prior apprehension is a much more common experience. In one survey, only fifteen out of forty-one doctors were happy to agree to being video-taped before the event, but thirty-four were happy to do it again after the event. Patients seem to forget that a camera is present and no-one in the Cardiff department requested scrubbing of a recorded consultation, despite the fact that all patients are invited to exercise this right after the session if they so wish.

However, these superficial statistics of acceptance do cover up a few important risks:

(a) Occasionally review sessions can become very destructive indeed and we have anecdotal evidence of doctors who have been severely shaken by the experience. This is most likely when a peer group fails to adhere to the ground-rules described above or when rather rigid norms of what is good consulting behaviour start to be applied by members of a group who are more experienced at video techniques than others.

(b) Confidentiality can be breached if strict codes of conduct are not observed. Tapes should only be viewed by people approved by the patient and doctor concerned.

(c) The focus of attention in a group is usually on the nature of doctor/patient communication and so discussion tends to revolve around the presenting problem (overt or covert). This in-depth analysis of the events seen on the tape is a narrow snapshot of both the living situation and the sequences revealed in the clinical record. Our experience is that it is quite difficult to get a video-view of wider issues or perceptions which are valued by doctor or patient. There is, therefore, a danger that analysis of the dynamics of communication will become a goal in itself and take investigation further and further from the realities of consultation events, which are not always revealed by looking at a single consultation.

In summary, in-depth consultation analysis using the video-tool gives a glimpse into the nature of a doctor-patient relationship. What is revealed is a real-life moment in time which may or may not be typical of the doctor's style and skills. Hence, like any snapshot it can reveal a weakness, a strength, a careless moment or an over-reaction under duress. Snapshots mean most to the actors in the picture and their power to influence self-perception, memories and behaviour is not in dispute. The abuse of snapshots is also a real possibility as a picture can be interpreted to modify the original meaning or to exaggerate a single aspect of the scene.

The video-taping of consultations has a place in medical education and research but our experience in Wales has led us to recognise that the fragmentary nature of the material must never be forgotten, particularly as there is some evidence to suggest that the most successful interviewers practice the greatest variation in style and pace. Our challenge is to encourage the majority of young doctors to be more flexible and to escape from the rigid moulds of their seniors, who, in Byrne and Long's words (1976), "display a remarkable inability to cope with anything but the most mechanical relationship with the patient".

The Consultation - Looking outward in Breadth

The consultation is the hub of primary care because it is here that processes are initiated which can be of momentous importance to the patient, the family and society at large. A wrong decision to refer may be very expensive for the individual or society, a missed opportunity for prevention or early diagnosis may seed later tragedy, and careless advice can result in unnecessary suffering. It is paradoxical that so many specialists like to view primary care as a simple filter which merely rations the flow of clientele into their selective care without questioning the principles which determine the nature and properties of that barrier. It is even more paradoxical that so many clinicians in primary care seem undisturbed by the evidence that a high proportion of their work concentrates on presenting problems and symptom relief alone.

Both the 'filter concept' and the 'episodic symptom relief' view of primary care debase the discipline and provide a cover for attitudes which conveniently deny the enormous potential which lies largely untapped in the vast majority of primary care encounters. One reason for under-valuing the potential in primary care is that we have failed to convince many influential people that primary care is more than a pot pourri of its component specialities. For example, many primary physicians seem content with massive duplication of effort over patient care: they will see a high proportion of their patients spontaneously every year but also send invitations to them to attend for cytology or immunization or blood pressure screening or developmental assessment etc. etc.; they will grumble about people who fail to comply with important therapy but let the same people pass through their hands with some trivial ailment, forgetting to review the more serious continuing problems; they will stick posters on their walls about protecting the doctor from trivial demands and yet practice trivial medicine by prescribing for every symptom.

It is for reasons such as these that there is a need to look at consultations in terms broader than their level of inter-personal communication. No consultation can be really effective if the level of communication is poor but likewise consultations become an expensive indulgence unless they are conducted with a broad view of goals and standards. The integration of prevention, cure and care is at the heart of modern primary care and the inclusion of social sciences is another requirement if primary care is to be relevant to the problems in society. How then can we begin to make these goals apply to the hurried activities which occur in the primary consulting room?

First we need an outline map which provides the surface features of our discipline. The outline we use in the Welsh National School of Medicine is the now familiar framework of the potential in every primary care conslutation (Figure 3). This has the merit of simplicity and so it can be memorised easily by the most junior of students or politicians. It also embraces four inter-related concepts

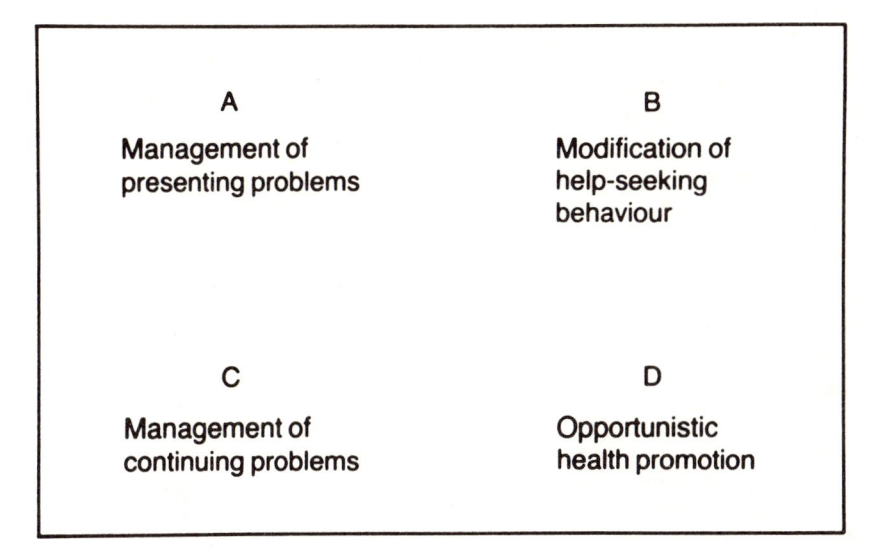

A Management of presenting problems	**B** Modification of help-seeking behaviour
C Management of continuing problems	**D** Opportunistic health promotion

Figure 3   The exceptional potential in every primary care consultation — an *aide memoire*

which need to be integrated into modern primary health care and it provides a framework upon which to hang detailed postgraduate study of our discipline. Most important of all, the framework provides a conceptual device which can be applied at every consultation. The fact that a minority of doctors do apply this framework at every consultation is not our immediate concern, because we are looking at potential rather than the status quo.

The framework of the exceptional potential in every consultation encourages clinicians to deal with the problems the patient presents, yet also to look beyond them to ask:

- Are there any continuing problems I should deal with while the patient is here?
- Why has the patient come to me at all(?) and what influence will my decisions/recommendations have on the patient's future expectations should similar clinical problems arise?
- Have I considered whether this patient is at risk due to poor life-style choices or a lack of preventive procedures?

This unashamedly patient-centred approach provides the broadest outline of an approach to every patient which uses the present to probe into the future and links curative thinking to preventive plans. It also brings the clinicians face to face with the consequences of their actions by emphasising the way in which people's expectations are moulded and the influence this may have on future help-seeking.

An unpleasant encounter may inhibit appropriate help-seeking in the future, whereas a careless clinical attitude may breed careless attitudes to the profession's services and inappropriate future demands.

Secondly, we must not confuse an outline framework with detailed mapping of every professional activity. The framework in Figure 3 is neither a detailed research instrument no a set of rules, tasks and skills. Its strength lies in its simple portrayal of the broad territory on which we can tread in each consultation. Having said that, I will be showing that it has considerable teaching and assessment power, despite its lack of specified detail in the diagram.

Thirdly, the concepts portrayed in the framework link the one-to-one clinical situation to the world outside the consulting room. No clinician can aim to apply this approach without facing the need for close collaboration with community nurses, educators, local counsellors, voluntary groups, community institutions, specialist teams etc. The doctor who wishes to beaver away in his own well-lined burrow without taking cognisance of the context in which he is working will perceive the framework as irrelevant. This reveals the power of this approach to clarify goals and to set the primary care services in their true colours.

What are the Consequences of Using the Framework?

When we started looking at primary consultations on video-tape, we tried to examine them in the light of the framework of potential and we quickly found the following:

(a) Most consultations appeared to be concerned with the presenting problem alone. Even the elderly with multiple problems appear to be dealt with episodically.

(b) It is impossible to rate a consultation using the four general areas in the framework because, by definition, the four areas overlap and embrace so many specific concepts that there is insufficient detail for acceptable reliability, sensitivity or specificity in rating methods.

(c) The framework approach to primary care is best revealed when good clinical records are combined with a glimpse of the exchanges in the consulting room. Video-tape alone is a poor indicator of the broad content of clinical care.

The value of the consulting framework is best revealed when patients' case-notes are discussed with the clinician involved. The notes reveal whether sequential consultations include more than episodic responses to isolated problems and the clinician can comment upon the unwritten goals or those forms of expression which are aide memoires but too subtle for the observer to follow alone. This approach also gives the clinician the opportunity to declare that whole areas of the framework are deliberately ignored:

> "I do not believe that it is a doctor's job to dabble in early diagnosis (screening) or prevention. We are here for cure and care."

This comment is helpful because it is obvious that the clinician is operating at a very different level from the one who said:

> "I use many patient contacts to explore risk factors in life-style and to perform/recommend simple screening tests but time is short and increasingly I send people through to our nurse for preventive procedures and discussion of major risks in their life-style."

The clinical record is probably the best single indicator of the breadth of a doctor's practice. The following are useful markers:

1. Markers to reveal that care of continuing problems is practiced effectively:

    (a) Clinical entries reflect interest in continuing problems (i.e. not only the presenting problem). The frequency of consulting obviously dilutes or concentrates this phenomenon so it has to be judged on several encounters.

    (b) Some form of problem list or summary of major/continuing problems appears in the records of patients with several important clinical events.

    (c) Plans are recorded which help a partner, trainee or locum understand the clinician's intentions for chronic or continuing problems.

    (d) Evidence that patients are involved in their own supervision, e.g. monitoring cards, repeat prescribing limits, shared-care records, self-help groups encouraged etc.

2. Markers that show whether help-seeking patterns are observed or acted upon.

    An awareness of the complex reasons why people consult doctors is the most important background knowledge in the area of help-seeking. A measure of application of this knowledge in practice would be the best indicator but this is not readily acquired from clinical records without discussing the issue with the clinician(s) concerned. The following are crude pointers:

    (a) Recording of problems which reflect awareness that distress is a frequent cause of consultation. 'Grief', 'unemployed', 'unhappy', 'lonely', 'angry' etc. are common examples.

(b) Regular use of therapy, other than procedures or prescriptions. 'Home remedies', 'counselling', 'relaxation exercises', 'volunteer group', 'social worker', 'youth group', 'minister' etc. reflect a breadth of community awareness and problem-solving perception.

(c) Comments which reveal concern/search for the roots of failed compliance, particularly the influence of family and friend networks.

3. Markers that reveal the degree to which opportunities are taken for early diagnosis or help with destructive lifestyles.

These are usually easy to observe because the clinical record should document entries such as:

Cervical cytology normal 1982
B.P. 120/30
Breast self-examination (B.S.E. - nurse)
Overweight (needs to lose 2 stone)
Smokes 40/day
High fat diet
Alcohol problem
Growing on 3rd percentile
Etc. etc.

However, the efficacy of such problem definitions will depend on there being some structure in the record so the items defined can be seen readily at a later date, then opportunistic health promotion becomes part of continuing care. The actions taken are beyond the scope of this paper but are dealt with elsewhere (Stott, 1983).

Summary

* Consultations can be examined in depth (e.g. video-analysis), or in breadth (e.g. by seeing whether clinical records reveal an orientation to more than episodic care). Both are perfectly valid ways of looking at the hub of primary care but both are necessary if balance is to be attained.

* Video-taped consultations provide sensitive material which has to be used with great care and understanding.

* The drive to classify styles is academically important but politically dangerous because the data is easily abused by those who are impressed by uniformity more than sensitivity.

* The framework of consultation potential is an outline map (surface features) of the tasks which face the clinician in primary care. It should be complimentary to more detailed classifications of tasks, skills and knowledge because it

helps to link the diversity of socio-medical theory to individual clinical practice. The outline map should become elaborated and coloured by individual training and experience into a colourful and fascinating discipline.

* The definition of markers which help to identify a breadth of approach to clinical primary care is an urgent and essential part of the discipline. We should be judged more by our breadth of approach and understanding than by the specialised knowledge we hold about individual disorders or problems.

ACKNOWLEDGEMENTS

The work described is a composite effort, involving many people in the Academic Department of General Practice in Wales. The Ely Primary Care Group and all those who participated in the studies deserve full recognition too. We are grateful to the Editors of the 'British Medical Journal', 'Patient Counselling and Health Education' and the Journal of the Royal College of General Practitioners for permission to reproduce the Figures 1, 2 and 3 respectively.

REFERENCES

Byrne, P. S. and Long, B. E. L., (1976) 'Doctors Talking to Patients,' H.M. Stationary Office.

Davis, R. H., Jenkins, M., Smail, S. A., Stott, N. C. H., Verby, J. and Wallace, B. B., (1980) 'Teaching with Audio-Visual Recordings of Consultations,' Journal of Royal College of General Practitioners, 30, 333-336.

Pendleton, D. A., Schofield, T. P. C., Tate, P. H. L. and Havelock, P. B., (1983) 'The Consultation: An Approach to Learning and Teaching,' Oxford University Press.

Stott, N. C. H. and Davis, R. H., (1979) 'The Exceptional Potential in Every Primary Health Care Consultation,' Journal of Royal College of General Practitioners, 29, 201-205.

Stott, N. C. H., (1983) 'Primary Health Care - Bridging the Gap between Theory and Practice,' Springer Verlag.

Verby, J. E., Holden, P., Davis, R. H., (1979) 'Peer Review of Consultation in Primary Care: The Use of Audio-Visual Recordings,' British Medical Journal, 1, 1686-1688.

Verby, J. E., Holden, P., Davis, R. H., (1980) 'A Study of Interviewing Skills in Trainee Assistants in General Practice,' Patient Counselling and Health Education, 2, 68-71.

18
Decision Analysis in General Practice

B.J. Essex

INTRODUCTION

Decisions made by general practitioners differ in many ways from those facing hospital doctors. The general practitioner deals with a wide range of unselected problems. Time is limited and there are many social and psychological factors that affect management.

Very little work has been done to explore how decisions are made in general practice. Emphasis is placed on what to do, not on why this decision was made. Medical students learn about decision-making in an unstructured way, largely through observation, and by emulating the thought processes they perceive to be used by their teachers. At present, few medical schools in the UK provide systematic instruction in decision-making skills. This is partly because of failure to recognise that there are critical skills, and partly because of lack of effective methods for training doctors to become good decision-makers. How relevant are some of the more recently developed techniques to decision-making in general practice?

Bayesian methods have been used to increase the accuracy of diagnostic decisions (Leaper et al., 1972). Good statistical data may support an effective Bayesian program where categories are small, overlapping and well defined. The inability to use qualitative knowledge limits the use of this approach in general practice, where problems are multidimensional and diagnostic categories are not mutually exclusive. Algorithmic methods are useful for some primary care tasks (Essex and Gosling, 1983) but are not appropriate in general practice. Where decisions are very complex, a doctor's reasoning style becomes less algorithmic, with qualitative judgmental knowledge becoming increasingly relevant (Elstein et al.,1978; Kassirer et al.,1978).

In the field of medical decision-making in the last 20 years, there has been progressively less dependence on observational data, and more emphasis on higher level knowledge. This includes 'judgmental' knowledge which reflects the experience and opinions of the expert. In the early 1970s, researchers began to investigate clinical applications of symbolic reasoning techniques drawn from the branch of computer science known as artificial intelligence. The field is well reviewed by Winston (1977). This work includes the development of programs that 'reason' about mineral exploration, organic chemistry and molecular biology as well as programs that generate theories from observations. This work has shown that qualitative experiential judgment can be codified in so-called 'rules of thumb' or 'heuristics', that focus on the most critical parts of the problem, and pursue a line of reasoning as opposed to a sequence of steps in a calculation.

Since decision-making in general practice also depends upon judgmental expertise, there must be rules or principles which operate even though these may not be recognised as such by the experienced doctor. The challenge is to identify what these are and how they influence our decisions. This is a most difficult area of research as the methodology needed to explore complex intellectual tasks is in its infancy. The methods out-lined below are experimental, empirical and limited. However, they are presented in the hope that critical analysis of different approaches will lead to more effective methods for undertaking research in this important field.

OBJECTIVES

The overall objective of a pilot research study started two years ago was to identify what kinds of decisions a general practitioner makes, and what influences these decisions. The aims were to:

Classify the types of decisions made in general practice

Identify the sequences in which decisions are made

Identify factors (variables) which affect decisions

Examine how these factors affect decisions

Define 'rules of thumb' that seemed to form the logical basis for decision-making.

Evaluate whether awareness of such rules increases the effectiveness of trainees' decision-making.

METHODOLOGY

The choice of methodology used in this pilot study was dictated by lack of resources, limited time available for each patient contact, and the difficulty of analysing one's own thought processes. Basic data

Figure 1: Decision Pathway

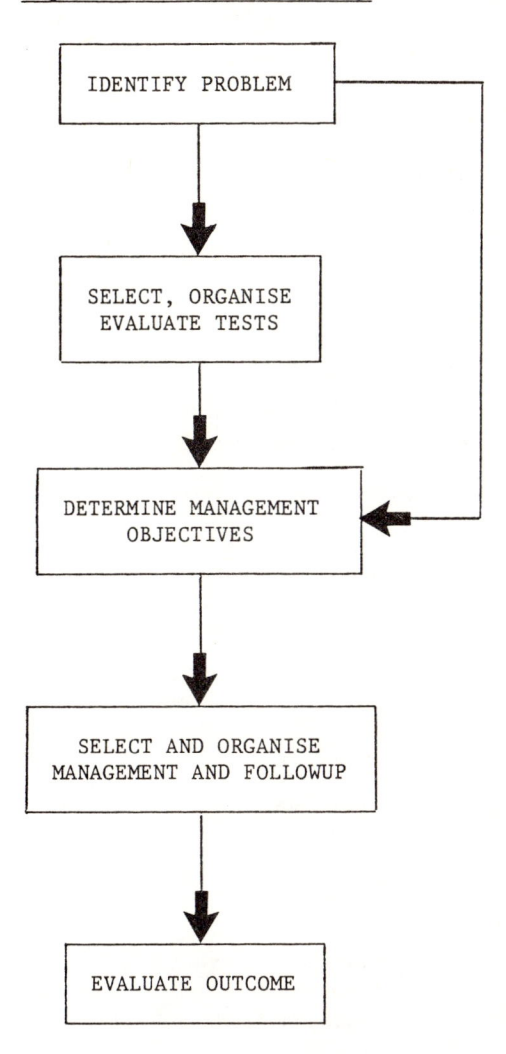

```
┌─────────────────────┐
│  IDENTIFY PROBLEM   │──────┐
└─────────┬───────────┘      │
          ▼                  │
┌─────────────────────┐      │
│  SELECT, ORGANISE   │      │
│   EVALUATE TESTS    │      │
└─────────┬───────────┘      │
          ▼                  │
┌─────────────────────┐      │
│ DETERMINE MANAGEMENT│◄─────┘
│     OBJECTIVES      │
└─────────┬───────────┘
          ▼
┌─────────────────────┐
│  SELECT AND ORGANISE│
│MANAGEMENT AND FOLLOWUP│
└─────────┬───────────┘
          ▼
┌─────────────────────┐
│  EVALUATE OUTCOME   │
└─────────────────────┘
```

were collected over 9 months. The following information was recorded on every patient contact I experienced during this time:

- the presenting problem and relevant observations

- what action was taken

- what factors affected my management decisions

- what rules, if any, seemed to form the logical basis for deciding to do A rather than B.

There were a total of 7522 patient contacts during this period. The stages of this study will now be outlined.

Classifying Decisions

All decisions relate to one of the five main objectives shown in Figure 1. The decisions relating to each task were then identified. For example, when evaluating outcomes, the general practitioner must decide:

- if evaluation is necessary

- who should undertake this task

- if follow-up evaluation is needed, how it should be organised

- what to tell patient about follow-up, possible complications of illness and treatment, and their management

- if patient defaults from follow-up, what to do, and how to organise it

- what observations to select to evaluate objective

- if outcome is successful, whether recurrence can be prevented, and if so, how

- if outcome is unsuccessful is this because of

    - diagnostic error

    - treatment being - inappropriate

                        - inadequate

                        - intolerable

                        - interacting with other drugs/disease

                        - incomprehensible to patient

- administrative error

- communication failure

- inappropriate objectives

- premature evaluation

- complications or new problem develops

- failure to prevent recurrence

- how unsuccessful outcome should be managed

Further analyses were done to classify the types of decisions made within each of these subgroups. This initial study resulted in the development of an empirical framework which enabled decisions to be readily classified, and their sequences to be identified.

Identifying Factors

Decisions in general practice are affected by many factors such as age, occupation, mental state etc. These also have to be identified and classified. To do this, the management of each problem was studied to identify the two or three factors which affected management decisions in each case. These data were recorded immediately after each patient contact. During the whole study period, a total of 93 factors were identified and classified as shown in Table 1. Although empirically derived, no factor affecting management decisions in general practice has been encountered that could not be placed in one of these groups.

Defining Rules

The hypotheses being explored here relate to whether or not there are rules which explain the relationship between factors and decisions. If two or three factors affect decisions about the management of a case, do these act independently, or are they dependent variables? What weight or priority ought to be attached to each one? In what way do these factors affect the decision process itself? To help to answer some of these questions any 'rule of thumb' which described how these factors affected the management decision was recorded. This was done immediately after each patient contact, as the initial impression was considered to be most important.

As a result of analysing many thousands of decisions a total of 324 'rules' were identified, which have varying degrees of applicability. These rules relate primarily to management, and to a far lesser extent to 'diagnosis'. They are basically of two types. A few relate to decisions about specific problems e.g. mental illness, coronary artery disease, diabetes etc. However, over 90% are not disease specific. They relate to a wide range of problems and therefore are more generally applicable. Some of these rules relate to the order in which things are done.

Examples of sequence rules are:

- "Decisions about management should be made after assessment of effects of problem on family"

Table 1: Factors Affecting Decisions

Health Problem

Aeteology
Differential diagnosis
Infectious possibility
Information accuracy
Natural history of illness
Objective findings
Probability of occurence
Problems – past or present
Seriousness/severity
Inbiased assessment
Urgency
Duration

Patient

Acceptability
Age
Appointment made with GP or not
At risk probability
Behaviour – addiction
          – breast feeding
          – defaulting
          – self discharge
          – violence
Compliance
Cultural factors
Disability

Doctor

Communication difficulties
Experience past
Expertise/skill – lack of
Ignorance
Knowledge
Mental state
Prejudices/values
Reaction to problem
Relationship with – other health personnel
                  – partners
                  – patient
                  – relatives
Uncertainty
Workload

Investigations

Indications
Reliability
Results

Resources

Allocation
Availability of – health personnel
                – other resources
                – skills

Expectations
Experience – past
Holiday – patient about to go on
Information – need for
Memory
Mental state
Nationality
Occupation
Pregnancy
Prejudices/values
Rights of
Sensitivities/allergies
Social/family circumstances
Treatment – previous responses
Lived in tropics

Family

Assessment – or problem by relatives
Family history
Information needs
Problem impact on
Requests
Responses

Other People

Effects of problem – on others in community
External pressures, requests
Person accompanying patient
Person who sent patient
Referral – direct from one clinic to another
Responses/opinions of – other doctors
                    – other people

Trainee/student present

Constraints
Hospital resources

Time factors

Day of week
Waiting list

Medico-legal

Confidentiality
Ethical factors
Legal factors
Responsibility

Management

Administrative factors
Contraindications
Indications for – continuing therapy
              – initiating therapy
Drugs – current administration
      – interactions
Economic factors
Effectiveness (benefits, advantages)
Errors
Geographical factors
Objectives
Option alternatives
Private practice
Side-effects (risks)
Practice policy/protocol

- "Decisions about management should be made after assessment of the family's ability to cope"

- "Decisions to assess compliance should precede decisions to evaluate outcome"

- "Decisions about long term place of care should be made after treatment of acute illness if present"

Some rules were initially disease specific. The case of the poorly controlled diabetic generated a rule relating to the need to assess compliance before changing diabetic medication. However, as this rule is equally applicable to many chronic diseases, its application is greater if changed to 'assess compliance before changing medication.'

Some rules describe the relationship between factors e.g. 'the patient's occupation may convert a non-urgent problem into an urgent one'. This rule recognizes a relationship between occupation and the urgency with which the problem is managed. The rule 'Perceptions of aetiology, urgency and severity have cultural determinants' identifies a relationship between cultural factors and three other variables. Other rules analyse urgency into its component parts and relates these to other factors e.g.:

"The method of communication with hospital is selected after assessing the urgency in psychological, social and physical terms"

Another rule analyses the assessment of urgency in more detail:

"Urgency is assessed by considering the natural history of the condition, and the probability of future complications as well as the severity of present disability"

Though derived from specific case studies, these rules all have a wide application. In fact there are a total of 37 rules that describe how this one factor, urgency, relates to other factors and affects a wide range of management decisions.

One of the most interesting findings was that most decisions had a rationale, the logical basis of which was not immediately apparent. However, after studying the management of each case, and the relevant factors which affected the decisions, it was possible to identify and define the 'rules of thumb' that seemed to be operating. These rules were derived from the study of a wide range of medical, social psychological and ethical problems presenting during the study period. Some of these rules have a time base, depending on currently accepted legal and ethical regulations. No attempt was made to be exhaustive as different rules might have been generated had more problems been studied.

Decision Analysis in General Practice

Relationship Between Decisions, Factors, Rules

The relationship between decisions, factors and rules is shown in the following case example:

An anxious Nigerian woman aged 24 comes to surgery. She requests referral for investigation of infertility. She has been married for 8 months and is not pregnant. She is worried about this. There is no past history of serious illness or pelvic infection, and she has not had any previous pregnancy.

What is your management?

Consider your management of this case and then ask yourself what factors affected your decisions. What rules describe how these factors affected your management? Try to answer these questions before reading on.

One of the most relevant questions to ask is 'What does your husband and his family think of all this?' The factors reflected in this inquiry include patient's mental state, and the impact of problem on the relatives. Other factors affecting management decisions here include cultural factors and the patient's perceptions of urgency. If you decided to reassure the patient that investigations were not needed at this time would the following rule have changed your management?

"Reassurance may be appropriate only after identifying the aetiology of anxiety."

The aetiology of anxiety in this case is itself related to cultural factors and a relevant rule is that:

"Cultural factors often determine the impact of a problem and the responses of patient and relatives"

The problem may have a non-urgent impact on the general practitioner but an urgent impact on the patient. The rule that reflects this states that:

"Perceptions of aetiology, urgency and severity often have cultural determinants"

The main decision to be made in this case is whether or not to accede to the patient's request for referral. The above analysis shows what factors affected the decision to refer the patient. The 'rules' indicate how these factors influenced the decision process itself.

One Factor, Many Rules - As the number of problems studied increased, it became possible to identify the many different kinds of decisions affected by a specific factor. For example, the waiting list affects decisions about acceptability, appointments, referrals, follow-up, investigations, etc. There are, therefore, many rules which show how waiting lists affect management decisions. With 93 factors affecting many different decisions, a precise index system is needed to identify all the rules relevant to a specific factor, and all the decisions affected by it.

One Rule, Many Factors - Just as one factor in different contexts generated many rules, so one rule may be based upon several factors. For example:

> The decision to advise without seeing the patient is based upon the likely differential diagnosis, the severity of illness, and the anxiety of patient and relatives.

This rule was derived from analysis of several cases where this was the critical decision being made. It relates to four different factors. Because of the complex relationship between decisions, factors and rules, each word has to be carefully selected and standardized to ensure it can be recalled when needed.

Making Connections - Most of the rules identified in this research project will be familiar to many doctors. They are not new and yet there are times when inappropriate decisions are made despite our awareness of the relevant rule involved. How often have we said 'I did X, yet I know Y should have been done first' or 'I just didn't think'? One explanation is that sometimes the right connections are not made. Knowledge of the rule is different from the ability to recall it when needed. Recalling a rule relevant to a specific management decision tests ability to make the right connections between a problem and the knowledge needed to solve it. From several hundred rules the one most relevant to this particular decision has to be selected. An index has been developed to explore how these connections are made. Such an index helps to:

- identify rules most relevant to any specific decision

- identify all the rules relating to any one factor

- identify sequence rules relating to the order in which decisions are made

- identify rules relating to management of specific illnesses

It then becomes possible to identify the rule relating to decisions about giving advice without first seeing the patient, by using the index and looking under management decisions, or advice, or differential diagnosis, or severity of illness or mental state.

Inexact Reasoning - Rules can be chained together in a way than enables some kind of logical deduction to be made. These rules can form a coherent explanation of inexact reasoning if the relevant ones are displayed in an appropriate sequence. Examine the following case:

An Asian mother brings her infant aged 5 months to the surgery with
a cough present for two days. Child looks fit, is afebrile and
chest is clear. ENT normal. There are no other abnormalities.
What do you do?

Before reading on, decide what your management would be. Now
consider the following rules:

- "Management objectives include prevention as well as cure"

- "Preventive medicine is often practised alongside identification and treatment of acute illnesses"

- "An important management objective is to prevent problems
  in at-risk patients"

- "An important management objective is to identify
  unvaccinated children who need to be immunized"

- "An important management objective is to prevent osteomalacia
  in high risk groups"

This case relates to decisions about management objectives. In
response to the question 'What am I trying to do?' these five rules
would be presented in the form of a chain in which broad concepts give
way to specific goals. As training advances, generation of the
concepts alone is often enough to enable the trainee to identify the
appropriate management.

It is difficult to link the rules together in a sequence that
initiates a reasoning process in the learner. Our knowledge itself is
incomplete and open ended, and new techniques need to be developed to
identify its inconsistencies and inadequacies. New methods are also
needed for the acquisition and integration of new facts and judgments.
The inexactness of our judgments and reasoning must somehow be
incorporated, perhaps by using some of the more recently developed
techniques which have been described (Shortliffe and Buchanan 1975).
In this decision support system rules can be linked to represent chains
of inexact reasoning. However, much more meticulous and
multi-disciplinary research is needed to develop effective ways of
doing this.

Priorities - One of the most difficult tasks in medicine is the
establishment of priorities. This is because these reflect our value
judgments and doctors and patients do not share the same values. When
a decision is affected by several factors, it is necessary to decide
what weight or priority to give to each. Legal and ethical factors,
including confidentiality, may have top priority, but the priority
given to other factors is more difficult to establish. For example,
management decisions about referral are affected by some or all of the
following factors: social and family circumstances, severity of
disability, GP's knowledge of other doctors, urgency, geographical

factors, acceptability, waiting lists, economic factors and hospital resources. In what order of priority would you place these factors?

There are many levels of complexity to the problem of priorities because these factors are not independent variables. For example, acceptability depends upon the patient's knowledge of other factors in the list. Moreover, priority given to these factors changes over time. Awareness of these interactions will affect the priorities given to these different variables. This in turn will affect the general practitioner's decision-making.

Evaluation

Many problems have been studied to identify what kinds of decisions are made, what factors affect them, and what decision-making rules seem to be operating. However, these findings have been generated by one person, and the question that must be asked is whether or not these rules lead to more effective decision-making by general practice trainees. To answer this question, an evaluation study needs to be done. Several steps are necessary to evaluate the effectiveness of this decision support system. The rules need to be revised by a group of experienced general practitioners. Test cases will be selected and a consensus of expert GP opinion will identify the decisions to be made, the relevant factors to be considered, and the optimal management of each problem. A scoring system will be developed and validated. Trainees' management decisions about each problem can then be rated before and after using the rules relevant to each case. Support is currently being sought to undertake this study.

DEVELOPMENT OF DECISION SUPPORT SYSTEM

If the results of this evaluation study show that trainees make significantly better decisions with the rules than without, the next step would be to develop a decision support system. This should be relevant to a wide range of decisions which the trainee has to make about medical, social, psychological and ethical problems encountered in general practice. It would be designed primarily for management, and would not provide specific diagnostic or therapeutic support, for which other decision aids are available. Through the analysis of management decisions about selected groups of cases, the trainee would learn to:

- classify the types of decisions which need to be made

- recognise the critical sequence in which decisions are made in general practice

- identify the most relevant factors that affect each decision in a specific case

- allocate appropriate priorities when one decision is affected by several factors

- use the index to identify the most useful rules that relate to the management of each case

- apply these rules whenever applicable to the management of other kinds of cases presented

The ultimate objective is to provide decision support whenever the trainee encounters difficulty with decisions about management of any new case encountered in daily practice. Such a decision support system should possess great flexibility and:

- be self-instructional

- be of use in surgery settings

- operate at different levels of sophistication and complexity depending on the needs of the user

- incorporate locally defined rules identified by GPs perhaps in conjunction with hospital doctors for management decisions of shared problems

- be updated, refined and revised when necessary

- be comprehensive enough to provide decision support for most problems encountered in general practice

A recurring observation made in the literature on computer based medical decision-making is that few, if any, systems have been effectively used outside of a research environment, even when performance is shown to be excellent. This may be because these systems do not enable the user to internalise the concepts and use them appropriately when needed. They encourage the user to be dependent rather than independent. As decision-making systems become more sophisticated, problems of acceptance will come to dominate this field. It is for this reason that acceptability and performance issues must be considered at the outset in a system's design because these considerations dictate the choice of methodology.

CONCLUSIONS

Even though this paper has outlined a pilot study prior to its evaluation, it is still possible to draw some conclusions about its findings and their implications.

The identification of a framework for analysing the types of decisions made in general practice and their sequences is useful. It enables an important source of error to be recognised. Management may be inappropriate, not because of lack of knowledge, but because of failure to realise that a specific decision must be made at this point in time. Without a way of examining the many different kinds of decisions made, and their sequences, it is difficult to demonstrate this source of error.

Before undertaking this research project, it would not have been possible to identify and categorise all of the factors that affect decisions in general practice. They have been grouped in a way that provides a comprehensive framework which is prerequisite for this kind of study. Attempts have already been made to identify how ethical factors affect doctor's decisions (Brody, 1981). This must now be done for the other 92 factors that affect management decisions in general practice.

Artificial intelligence researchers have developed promising methods for handling concurrent diseases (Pople, 1977,; Weiss, et al., 1978), assessing time courses of diseases, and for acquiring structured knowledge from the experts. These programs all stress the need to understand underlying concepts. This search for the conceptual basis of decision-making in general practice has resulted in the definition of many 'rules of thumb'. These were identified by analysis of individual cases and this pragmatic approach seemed appropriate. However, the study shows that expert system techniques can be used to identify decision processes in general practice. When criteria for decision-making become explicit, much that is uncertain, irrational and illogical becomes apparent. These areas deserve the closest study.

As a result of this pilot study it becomes feasible to audit decision-making in general practice. The criteria for 'good' decision-making include the ability to:

- identify all relevant decisions that need to be made

- make decisions in the correct order

- select relevant factors

- give each factor its due priority

- consider relevant rules

- take appropriate, cost-effective and acceptable action

However, we do not know whether decisions based on these considerations lead to more effective management. The next phase of this research study will attempt to answer the following questions:

- To what extent do other doctors agree with these rules?

- How valid are they?

- How can these rules be chained together to present inexact reasoning processes?

- Can knowledge of these decision pathways, factors and rules be used to increase trainees' decision-making skills?

We are trying to encode and use expert knowledge which cannot be obtained from data banks or literature reviews. Here, an understanding of reasoning processes and strategies themselves is essential, yet these have never been explicitly represented. What is now needed is a multidisciplinary approach to develop new methods which will have to be rigorously evaluated. The real demystification of medicine will not occur until doctors understand how they make complex decisions, and are able to share this knowledge with others.

REFERENCES

Brody, H., (1981). Ethical Decisions in Medicine. Little, Brown and Company, Boston.

Davis, R. (1977). Interactive Transfer of Expertise. Acquisition of New Inference Rules. In Proceedings of 5th International Joint Conference on Artificial Intelligence (Cambridge, MA).

Elstein, A. S., Shulmman, L. S., Sprafka, S. A. (1978). Medical Problem-solving. An Analysis of Clinical Reasoning. Cambridge, MA, Harvard University Press.

Essex, B. J., Gosling, H. (1983). An Algorithmic Method for Management of Mental Health Problems in Developing Countries. British Journal of Psychiatry, 143, pp 451-459.

Kassirer, J. P., Gorry, G. A. (1978). Clinical Problem-solving: A Behavioural Analysis. Annual of International Medicine, 89, pp. 245-255.

Leaper, D. J., Horrocks, J. C., Staniland, J. R., de Dombal, F. T. (1972). Computer Assisted Diagnosis of Abdominal Pain using Estimates Provided by Clinicians. British Medical Journal, 4, pp. 350-354.

Pople, H. (1977). The Formation of Composite Hypotheses in Diagnostic Problem-solving: An Exercise in Synthetic Reasoning. Proceedings of 5th International Conference on Artificial Intelligence, Cambridge, MA, pp. 1030-1037.

Shortliffe, E. H., Buchanan, B. G. (1975). A Model of Inexact Reasoning in Medicine. Mathematical Biosciences, 23, pp. 351-379.

Weiss, S. M., Kulikowski, C. A., Amarel, S., Safir, A., (1978). A Model-Based Method for Computer-Aided Medical Decision-Making. Artificial Intelligence, 11, pp. 145-172.

Winston, P. H. (1977). *Artificial Intelligence.* Reading, MA, Addison Wesley.

19
Discussion of the Papers by Stott and Essex

Mike A. Pringle

This session started with Dr Stott enlarging on his paper and reinforcing his plea for students to be taught the wider aspects of consultation technique. He wished students to be encouraged to learn the art of accurate observation and to include wider, prevention orientated, care within the consultation.

This lack of accent on the diagnostic decision process itself was clarified by questions concerning how a student can be taught to 'control' patients with patient-centred consultations. The avoidance of 'rambling' and problem evasion were highlighted.

Evidence to support video camera use was presented, showing that videotaping had no effect on patient anxiety as compared to controls, whereas a doctor observer was shown to be a stimulator of patient anxiety.

However, most discussion centred on the 'registrars' study. It became apparent that the registrars were in fact trainees in general practice in the last six months of their three year course. There was a desire to see a duplication of these results, especially in regard to the deteriorating performance of the 'controls'.

Collaborative evidence was volunteered, partly from equivalent studies, and from the 'de-skilling' which occurs in the process of learning new tasks. Anecdotal evidence for the stress implicit in trainees in their early days in practice was produced from several participants from the U.S. and Canada.

This was felt to be largely due to the new medical conditions being seen, which do not necessarily match the standard hospital descriptions, and the new method of working. Partly this can be seen as the process towards patient-centred care.

Increasing skills through video tapes did, of course, lengthen consultation duration, but there was speculation that this time might be saved in the long run through improved achievement in the consultation.

We were pleased to learn that these self-same 'registrars' were being re-evaluated in their practices now, which should supply further information on the long term effect of videotape education. We were cautioned, however, against reading too much into these results which were not statistically significant.

The issues of the effect of student and junior doctor consultations on the patients was raised, but unfortunately asking patients' opinion after their consultation provided bland platitudes. It was observed that matching patient expectation before consultation with their satisfaction afterwards would be more likely to be useful. Discussion of Dr. Stott's paper finished on a cautionary note concerning the dangers of introducing computerised decision support before defining the principles of our discipline - which could lead to fragmentation of the roles of the doctors.

Dr. Essex presented his paper, and it was quickly seen as a sound first step towards creating a rule system applicable to General Practice decision-making support aids. The computer scientists present welcomed this initiative, and felt it complemented their current hospital based efforts.

There was considerable controversy concerning validation of the rules in Dr. Essex's system. Some felt that they should be universal, with the capacity for individual alterations; others that it should only be accurate for Dr. Essex; still others wanted validation to be on the basis of assessing whether, retrospectively, the rule predicted the outcome.

The consensus was that these rules were a useful tool for demonstrating errors in process and were as thus a valuable teaching aid. This overcame the problems concerning inter-doctor agreement on the rating of decisions, since the learning criteria were subjective for that student. The point was made that this system was not designed to look at diagnosis, or management selection, but purely at the area exemplified by: "I know what I have done, but why did I do it?" Proliferation of rules was prevented by keeping to the high non-specific level, with low level specific rules minimised.

Dr Essex said that he had found the process of formulating his rules illuminating and educational, and there was much discussion concerning whether this was the real benefit, and whether all users of the system might benefit as much from selecting their own rules as from using the system itself.

It was also observed that the rule structure for each doctor could be used to define just how patient-centred or doctor-centred that G.P. was.

In summary, these two papers provoked a lively and stimulating debate and left an impression that they both dealt with the realities and vagaries of general practice to a degree that many concepts or theories do not.

20
A Computer-assisted Diagnostic Decision System for Dyspepsia

R.P. Knill-Jones, W.M. Dunwoodie and G.P. Crean

INTRODUCTION

Dyspepsia is a common problem in the community and a frequent reason for attendance at a G.P.'s surgery. A proportion of patients are referred to hospital for further investigations, many of which prove to be negative. It has been argued that many of the inappropriate investigations could be avoided given more accurate or more confident diagnoses made when the patient first presents to a doctor (BMJ, 1978). Availability of simple diagnostic aids might help towards this general aim. However these aids take a considerable amount of time and work to develop, and require extensive evaluation before being acceptable for routine use.

This paper is in two parts - first we briefly summarise 10 years' work in Glasgow directed towards an investigation of dyspepsia with the long-term aim of developing simple decision-aids. The problem was deliberately chosen because it was a difficult one, in contrast to the better defined areas previously used for developing decision aids. For example:- Professor Sir Edward Wayne and his Thyroid Index, Professor T.R Taylor on round shadows on thyroid 'lumps', Tim de Dombal on acute abdominal pain, Dr A Alperovitch on round shadows on the chest x-ray and one of the current authors on jaundice diagnosis. Dyspepsia is difficult because it comprises a wide range of diseases, includes a large component of non-organic disease, and even after a full investigation a patient may be found to have incomplete evidence for one diagnosis or may even have evidence for several diagnoses. Secondly we discuss the general problem of evaluation of a decision aid and present some initial evaluations of the dyspepsia system. These were sufficiently encouraging to set up a randomised controlled trial of its effect in general practice; the method for this is given in detail.

History-taking and Computer Interrogation

One characteristic of "dyspepsia" is that the history is of great importance. Information from the patient can of course be obtained by a doctor in the usual way. However several studies have shown considerable differences when histories are taken in this way by different doctors from the same patient. Attempts to reduce this 'observer error' involved much discussion in the early years of the project. Eventually definitions of each symptom in the history were agreed. Work had also started in trying to standardise the process by presenting the questions to the patient on a teletype and using a computer to direct the consultation process. This was found to be acceptable to patients and also to have a good reproducibility (Card et al, 1974., Lucas et al, 1976). The process of automating the information-gathering component of the clinical history does not result in "history-taking" in the normal clinical sense - after all most of the non-verbal clues will be missed by such a device! The one non-verbal clue that can be measured during computer-based questioning is the patients' reaction time to each question. Symptoms recognised by the patient tend to produce a much quicker response than questions about symptoms which he has never experienced. The process is best regarded as 'interrogation' (Card & Lucas, 1981) and not as "history-taking". Careful attention to the use of simple words and phrasing was found to help in patient acceptability and comprehension.

The current system works on an Apple computer with a special keyboard containing buttons marked 'Yes', 'No', and 'Don't understand'. The 'Yes' and 'No' buttons can be qualified by 'Certainly', 'Probably' and 'Possibly'. (See Fig.1) There is also a 'Go Back' button to allow a patient to correct a response. A similar system also runs on a PDP 11/34; in this system a further refinement is that the speed of the interview is automatically varied according to the patients' verbal reading ability; this limited interaction with particular characteristics of individual patients could be further

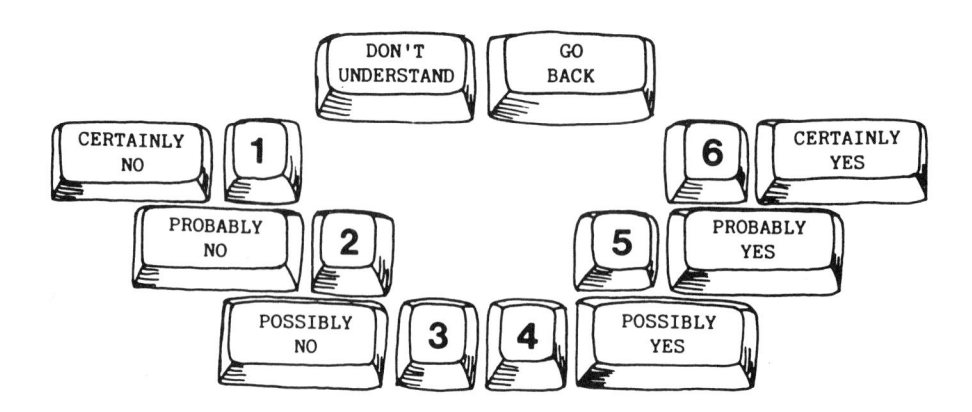

FIGURE 1

developed, making the device a little more intelligent than the simplest of systems.

Dyspepsia Data base

While developments of the patient-computer interface continued steadily, clinical effort went into the collection of data using standard proformas which included clear definitions of each symptom. There are now some 1200 patients in the data base, which includes items from the history, examination, sigmoidoscopy, Middlesex Hospital Questionnaire; also results from haematological and biochemical investigation together with standardised reports from endoscopy and radiology which were carried out 'blind' - that is without clinical information unless specially requested.

Clinicians recorded their initial clinical diagnoses - in terms of the probability that a disease was present - at the time of first patient contact; this information allowed 'retrospective' evaluation of the diagnostic aid in comparison to these clinical diagnoses.

Table 1: Primary Diagnosis in 1176 patients. Broad Classification

	N	%
Simple oesophageal disease	45	3.8
Complicated oesophageal disease	63*	5.4
Duodenal ulcer disease	330	28.1
Gastric ulcer disease	74*	6.3
Irritable bowel syndrome	177	15.0
Organic bowel disease	63*	5.4
Gallstones	50*	4.2
Alcohol-induced dyspepsia	48	4.1
Gastric cancer	32*	2.7
Non organic disease	294	25.0
TOTAL	1176	

*These 282 patients should normally be managed by referral for hospital investigation. The remaining patients could initially be managed in general practice.

Final diagnoses were eventually agreed for 1176 of the 1200 cases - 24 (2.0%) could not have a final diagnosis made - usually because of incomplete information and failure of follow up. The final diagnosis was made at least six months after the patient first presented using information from investigations, response to treatment and peer review if necessary. Up to three G.I. diagnoses were recorded, and each was qualified by 'Certain', 'Probable' or 'Possible'. The breakdown is given below and refers to the Primary or first diagnosis; the additional diagnoses are not discussed in this paper but contribute to the data used by the decision aid. A broad classification appropriate for initial management of the patient is given, this being appropriate for the management-orientated decisions made in a General Practice setting. A more detailed diagnostic classification relevant to specialist practice is also available; for example of the 74 cases of gastric ulcer disease 68 had an ulcer demonstrated and six had only evidence of an ulcer scar.

Development of a decision aid

The problem now was to bring together the computer interview and the data base so that a diagnostic aid could be developed. Many such aids have depended on the simple procedure of using Bayes Theorem with assumption of independence of symptoms within the disease classes. This method is inappropriate for dyspepsia because of multiple final diagnoses and of strong dependence between many of the symptoms. The statistical method has be described in detail and is based on an application of Logistic Discrimination (Spiegelhalter & Knill-Jones, 1984). The paper includes an extensive review of 'expert systems' and the ways in which that approach differs from the conventional statistical one used here. The principles of the method and the results of initial evaluations of the decision aid are given below.

OUTLINE OF STATISTICAL METHODS

Simple techniques of statistical diagnosis do not work well in dyspepsia because their basic assumptions do not hold - 33% of patients with dyspepsia have at least two diagnoses, and the symptoms of dyspepsia are highly interdependent; furthermore 5% of patients have three diagnoses.

The solution adapted for the Diagnostic Decision System was to consider each possible disease in turn and to use Logistic Discrimination to differentiate between "presence of the disease" and "absence of the disease".

The principle underlying the method is that for each disease the data base is searched for those symptoms which discriminate best. The method allows dependent symptoms to be eliminated, for example "Wind" and "Bloating" tend to be closely related, or "dependent" symptoms, only one should be included. Usually only a few symptoms are

A Computer-assisted Diagnostic Decision System for Dyspepsia   207

necessary to give very good discrimination, and all other symptoms then provide no significant increase in discriminating power.

Let us consider, an an example, the problem of Gallstones causing dyspepsia. It can be shown that seven symptoms provide excellent discrimination. The weights, or "scores" associated with presence or absence of each of these symptoms are shown in Table 2.

Table 2: Symptoms and their weights used in the diagnosis of Gallstones

INDICANT	INDICANT STATE AND ITS ASSOCIATED SCORE:	
Length of history:	Longer than one year:	-44
	Between 6 months and 1 year:	9
	Less than 6 months	77
Pain in Right Hypochondrium:	Absent:	-53
	Present:	77
Pain severe enough to seek emergency help:	No	-43
	Yes	68
Radiation of Pain:	None:	-38
	To Back:	16
	To Shoulder Tip:	129
Attacks of Pain:	Absent:	-141
	Present:	177
For those with attacks of pain		
Enumeration of attacks	Absent:	-141
	Present:	63
Restlessness	Absent:	-141
	Present:	31

A high score indicates that the symptom is strongly in favour of the diagnosis (eg. a history of less than six months scores +77), whereas a negative score is against the diagnosis (eg. inability to enumerate attacks of pain scores -141).

The most informative symptoms can easily be seen from such tables. Those with the biggest range of scores provide the most information. In the given example, "attacks of pain" is the most informative symptom with a range of scores of 318. These scores also show at a glance which symptoms are in favour of a diagnosis and which are against.

The scores are simple to use. If a patient has a short history, has no attacks of pain but has Right Hypochondrial pain which radiates to the shoulder tip, his score is 77 - 141 +77 + 129 = +142. To obtain the probability of Gallstones from this score it is first necessary to subtract a constant which represents the prior incidence of the disease (for Gallstones 300), giving a total score of -158. This is then converted to a probability (by calculation or by reference to a table or graph), in this instance 0.17. The same score may be used in a different population of patients by changing the one score which reflects the incidence of the disease in the new population.

APPLICATION OF THE STATISTICAL MODEL

In principle, symptom 'scores' can be made widely available on cards, in booklets, etc., and for the whole dyspepsia system only 65 symptoms need to be elicited and 11 simple calculations done. It is not essential to have a computer for this task. However an alternative solution is to elicit the symptoms directly from the patient by computer interviewing, enabling the calculations and report generation to be done automatically, and relieve medical staff from the tedium (and discipline) of filling in questionnaires.

EVALUATION OF THE SYSTEM

The evaluation of such a system in relation to its effect on health care is complex. Some of the difficulties can be illustrated by another example.

Suppose that a probability of 0.9 was calculated for Simple Oesophageal Disease and a probability also of 0.9 was calculated for Duodenal Ulcer Disease for the same patient. In this case the probabilities clearly add up to more than 1.0 and the obvious interpretation is the patient may have both diseases. While this is entirely sensible from a clinical viewpoint, the evaluation of decision-aids making such suggestions is complex.

In the past, most statistical models for diagnosis have been assessed simply on their ability to calculate accurately one diagnosis, the 'diagnosis' being that with the highest probability. This was done for dyspepsia on a prospective series of 150 patients interviewed by computer. The highest probability given by the computer to any diagnosis was called the "first" diagnosis, and these diagnoses were compared with the "final" diagnoses. In these 150 patients, the primary final diagnosis was given the highest probability in 37% of patients, was in the highest two in 57%, and in the highest 3 in 68%. The corresponding figures for the consultant's diagnoses at first interview were 61%, 74% and 78%.

Such a method does not indicate to what extent decisions made about management might be correct, and these might often be unrelated to the order of calculated probabilities. As will be seen below the computer suggestions were comparable to those made by Consultants on the same 150 patients. In the example given above it would be acceptable to treat the patient both for Duodenal Ulcer Disease and Simple Oesophageal Disease without further investigation, as both were highly likely (odds of 9 to 1 on) to be present.

On the other hand, suppose that the same patient also had a probability of Gastric Carcinoma calculated at 0.2. The right decision would then be quite different. Endoscopy would be essential to establish or rule out this diagnosis.

Evaluation therefore has to be done in terms of decisions made rather than diagnostic accuracy. This is completely appropriate given that it is management at the General Practitioner/hospital interface which is being considered. The managements suggested by the system include immediate referral to hospital services, referral for investigations, and a range of treatment regimes. The decision rules for the various suggested managements contain both diagnostic and management information. They are arranged in hierarchy of importance, thus the first rule is: "Possibly Gastric Carcinoma: Refer immediately to G.I. Clinic".

PRELIMINARY EVALUATION OF SYMPTOM SCORES (RETROSPECTIVE TRIAL)

The symptom scores were initially devised using a set of 819 patients and the first validation exercise was then done on 100 different cases. The data from which diagnostic and management suggestions were calculated for these 100 was the history data collected by the Consultants using the same structured questionary as had been used in the collection of the original data base.

These 100 cases comprised those for whom it had taken some time to arrive at a final diagnosis; they were more 'difficult' cases than a truly random or consecutive series.

In spite of this, the results of this preliminary validation experiment were encouraging. The management suggestions made by the model can be grouped in three broadly comparable sets of actions; first referral to hospital gastrointestinal services, second, referral for X-ray investigation, and third, treatment by the General Practitioner himself. In this series of 100 patients, all of whom had already been referred to hospital by their General Practitioners, the computer would have referred only 47% and requested X-rays in 26%, compared with the Consultants who would have referred 26% and X-rayed 9%. The remaining cases would all have had treatments recommended, 63% of those recommended by the computer being "appropriate" compared with 68% of those recommended by the Consultants.

There were three notable mistakes made by the Consultants and three made by the computer, both being wrong simultaneously about one patient. A notable mistake occurs when treatment is recommended for a patient with serious organic disease for which referral to a Gastrointestinal Centre would be the best management decision.

PROSPECTIVE TRIALS USING COMPUTER INTERVIEWS

Following this preliminary evaluation using data collected by doctors, two truly prospective trials using data obtained by computer interview were done. In each of these trials, the management decisions suggested by the computer systems are compared with those that would have been suggested by the consultant gastroenterologist on the first interview of the patients. This is done for three groups of patients: First, those for whom the final diagnosis would have demanded referral to hospital. Second, those for whom the final diagnosis was of organic disease which could be treated without referral. Third, those for whom the final diagnosis was of a non-organic cause for their dyspepsia.

(Note. In the tables, "Treat approp." means "Treat appropriately", and "Treat not approp." means "Treat inappropriately". "No Decision" means that the consultant was unable to give an independent opinion as the diagnosis may already have been established).

PROSPECTIVE TRIAL NUMBER 1:

Evaluation in an outpatient clinic, Southern General Hospital.

A consecutive series of 150 patients attending an outpatient clinic were interviewed by the computer as well as by a consultant. The management that would have been suggested by the computer was compared to that suggested by the Consultants at their 'first interview'.

Tables 3, 4, and 5 show these comparisons for three groups of patients, grouped according to their final diagnoses: for those who should have been referred, those who had organic disease which could have been treated in General Practice, and those with non-organic causes of their dyspepsia.

The computer is 'tuned' to perform well with this group and err on the safe side. The only reason that two mistakes (see row labelled "Treat not approp" in Table 3) were made by the computer is that a tentative diagnosis of an alcohol problem was made for both patients where a diagnosis of "Insufficient Evidence" would have been correct. One of these patients had a benign gastric ulcer and the other a carcinoma of the caecum. The Consultants made 5 notable mistakes, (see column labelled "Treat not. approp." in Table 3), inappropriately

Table 3: Patients who should have been referred to hospital

Consultant's Decision at First Interview:

		Refer	X-Ray	Treat approp.	Treat not approp.	No Independent Decision	Total
Computer System Decision	Refer	24	-	-	3	7	34
	X-Ray	2	-	-	2	4	8
	Treat approp.	-	-	-	-	-	-
	Treat not approp.	1	-	-	-	1	2
	Total	27	-	-	5	12	44

Table 4: Patients with organic disease who need not be referred

Consultant's Decision at First Interview:

		Refer	X-Ray	Treat approp.	Treat not approp.	No Independent Decision	Total
Computer System Decision	Refer	14	1	13	7	1	36
	X-Ray	2	1	6	2	4	15
	Treat approp.	1	-	8	1	4	14
	Treat not approp.	2	-	2	3	1	8
	Total	19	2	29	13	10	73

Table 5: Patients with no organic disease

Consultant's Decision at First Interview:

		Refer	X-Ray	Treat approp.	Treat not approp.	No Independent Decision	Total
Computer System Decision	Refer	7	-	3	5	-	15
	X-Ray	-	-	1	2	-	3
	Treat approp.	1	1	1	2	3	8
	Treat not approp.	-	-	3	3	1	7
	Total	8	1	8	12	4	33

treating and not referring one patient with a gastric carcinoma, one with a benign gastric ulcer, one with Gallstones, one with Crohn's Disease, and one with "Organic Symptoms". This may indicate a tendency by the Consultants to take more 'risks' than the general practitioners who had referred the patients in the first place.

The computer referred 49% of the patients in this group and requested X-ray on a further 21%. The Consultants did much better, referring only 30% (19/63) and requesting X-rays in only 3%. Of those patients who would have been recommended for treatment, the computer would have been correct about the choice of treatment for 64% (14/22) of patients compared with the Consultant's 69% (29/42).

In this final group, the computer again would have recommended fewer (45%) treatments than the Consultants (69%). Of these, the computer would have recommended correct treatment for 53% compared with the Consultant's 40%.

Thus over the whole series, the computer would have referred 57%, requested X-ray for 17%, and treated 26%, while making two mistakes. The Consultants would have referred 44%, requested X-ray for 2%, and treatment 54%, while making five notable mistakes. The local General Practitioners had referred 100%.

PROSPECTIVE TRIAL NUMBER 2:

Evaluation in Monklands District General Hospital, Airdrie.

A consecutive series of 30 patients referred to medical and surgical outpatient clinics were interviewed by a consultant who completed a "diagnosis at first interview" and then requested a computer interview. Final diagnoses were established when all investigations had been completed and some response to treatment observed. (Only 30 such case were available at the time of analysis).

Again, managements suggested by the Consultants at first interview and those suggested by the computer were compared in three groups of patients.

The computer and the Consultants performed very similarly in the group of patients with organic disease who need not be referred; both would have recommended treatment for approximately 40% of patients, nearly all of which would have been correct treatments.

Over the whole series of patients, the computer would have referred 53% of patients, requested X-ray for 17%, and recommended treatment for 30%, while making one mistake - a history of pain but not of attacks of pain, was obtained in a patient with cholelithiasis. The Consultants would have referred only 26%, requested X-ray for 37%, and recommended treatment for 37%, while making no notable mistakes.

CONCLUSION OF PRELIMINARY EXAMINATION

At the current stage of development, the use of the Diagnostic Decision System for Dyspepsia in primary care might potentially save 43% of referrals to hospital outpatient clinics. Considering the mistakes made by the computer and made by the Consultants in the two prospective trials, it is reasonable to expect no fall in the standard of health care but possibly a slight increase. On this basis it was felt that it would be ethically acceptable to mount a trial in general practice.

A Computer-assisted Diagnostic Decision System for Dyspepsia

EVALUATION WITHIN THE COMMUNITY

Assessment of Computer-assisted diagnostic aid for dyspepsia in General Practice

As indicated above we thought that it would be of great interest to see whether a decision aid developed within the hospital service could contribute to the care of dyspeptic patients when they are seen initially by their family doctors. A project was set up in Govan Health Centre, Glasgow, to examine the impact such a machine might have. The first patient was referred in July 1982 and to date 360 patients have been seen.

Aims

The questions to be answered by this project are as follows:

1. Is a computer-assisted diagnostic system which interviews patients and makes suggestions about management acceptable to patients and doctors in General Practice?

2. Does the use of the computer system result in lower costs to the National Health Service?

3. Does the use of the computer system alter the management, within General Practice, of patients with dyspepsia?

Evaluation of a decision aid raises complex problems as indicated earlier and we first consider the features of current management which affect any assessment of the device in a general practice setting.

Mechanics of Current Management

The area of gastrointestinal symptoms in which we currently work is one both of considerable economic importance and of significant patient morbidity. It was noted in the introduction that G.I. symptoms are prevalent in the community. For example, a symptom prevalence survey carried out in Glasgow found that nausea, retching, and vomiting occurred in 8.8% of the sample in a two week period prior to the survey, heartburn or indigestion in 14.8% and abdominal pain or a bowel upset in 12.0% (Hannay, 1978). Furthermore, in 1978/79 11 million working days for men were lost from digestive diseases. 2.7 million were lost for women over the same period (Social Security Statistics 1980).

Following the development of symptoms, patients may either self-treat or present to their family doctor. At this initial contact the G.P. will attempt to formulate some working diagnostic tag. Sometimes the history alone may be sufficient, for example, where someone presents with simple indigestion or with well-defined symptoms such as occur in gastroenteritis where there may also be a history of eating a suspect meat pie! When the history is not sufficient either referral or investigation, or both, may be required. It is this area of investigation and referral wherein lies the principal area of cost to the NHS in terms of resources and to the patient in terms of time off work and protracted morbidity until specific appropriate therapy is started.

The computer based decision-aid described in the first section may offer a means of short-circuiting this system. Figure 2 outlines the flow of patients through the system and indicates where any potentially beneficial effect might occur - reducing referral and investigation may lead to quicker investigation of effective 'treatment' (used in a broad sense in which drug therapy is only a part).

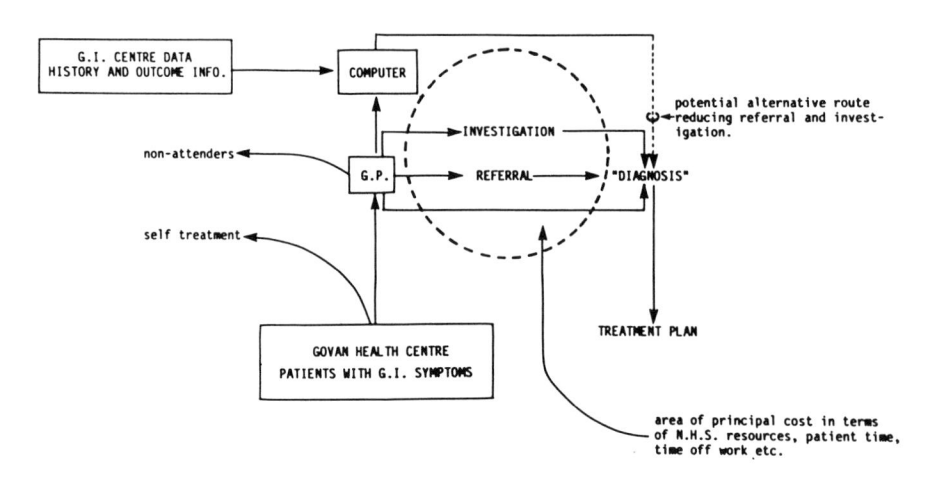

FIGURE 2

Setting in the Community

The questionnaire and underlying data has been generated over several years using patients presenting to the Southern General Hospital in Glasgow. It is valuable, therefore, when evaluating the system at this stage that the General Practitioners who are now using it are all located within the catchment area of the Southern General Hospital - all are in the South-West of Glasgow. This means that the geographical, social structure and clinical characteristics of the group upon whom the dyspepsia data is based is similar to the group who will be using the machine in primary care.

A Computer-assisted Diagnostic Decision System for Dyspepsia

Computer Output

Initially the output from the machine merely provided a simple list including one, two or three diagnostic statements with suggested actions and a list of G.I. illnesses together with the probability predicted for each. A recent example is given in Table 6.

Obviously this required modification, but in a direction which reflected the needs of the general practitioners who would be using the system. Opinions were sought from local participating General Practitioners and as expected there was a general feeling that the statements provided were too bald and gave neither reasons nor justifications for the diagnoses put forward. There was clearly need for compromise whereby opinion would be provided in an easily digested form complete with the indications which had led to the 'diagnoses' and yet would not be such a lengthy or complicated document that it would not be read. The output was therefore modified and divided into

TABLE 6

PATIENT'S IDENTIFICATION: 1   DATE OF COMPUTER INTERVIEW: 03-07-84

DIAGNOSTIC STATEMENT APPROPRIATE	SUGGESTED ACTIONS
1 Possibly Gastric Cancer:	Refer to Hospital G.I. Service
5 Possibly Severe Oesophageal Disease:	Refer to Hospital G.I. Service

DISEASE	P	ODDS
Severe Oesophageal Disease	.4717	1 TO ONE AGAINST
Gastric Carcinoma	.387	2 TO ONE AGAINST
Duodenal Ulcer Disease	.2355	3 TO ONE AGAINST
Insufficient Evidence	.1597	5 TO ONE AGAINST
Simple Oesophageal Disease	.1555	5 TO ONE AGAINST
Organic Bowel Disease	.0922	10 TO ONE AGAINST
Irritable Bowel Syndrome	.0571	17 TO ONE AGAINST
Gastric Ulcer Disease	.0515	18 TO ONE AGAINST
Nervous Dyspepsia	.0452	21 TO ONE AGAINST
Progressive Alcohol Problem	.0104	96 TO ONE AGAINST
Cholelithiasis	.0041	242 TO ONE AGAINST

three separate sheets. The first presents the individual decisions together with a list of symptoms which point to the diagnosis and symtoms which are absent and might point away from the diagnosis: in essence a 'balance sheet' of the evidence for and against the hypothesis.

The example in Table 7 is part of the printout for the patient in the previous table. The weight of evidence for the diagnosis is given to the left of each symptom. For example in the upper section which explains the probability of 0.39 for Gastric Cancer there are four

Table 7

First part of output

GLADYS

RECOMMENDED ACTIONS, DIAGNOSES, AND SYMPTOMS

DECISION 1   Possibly Gastric Cancer: Refer to Hospital G.I. Service

    DIAGNOSIS: Gastric Carcinoma   P = .39   (2 to ONE AGAINST)

Symptoms for the Diagnosis   Symptoms against the Diagnosis
    PRESENT
(225) Age > 55
(138) Length of history < 1 year
(100) Lost over half stone in last 6 months
(63) Early repletion

DECISION 2   Possibly Severe Oesophageal Disease: Refer to Hospital G.I. Service

    DIAGNOSIS: Severe Oseophageal Disease   P = .47   (EVENS)

Symptoms for the Diagnosis   Symptoms against the Diagnosis

    PRESENT
(128) Length of history < 1 year   (-92) No dysphagia
(62) Never experiences 'bloating'   (-68) Female
(56) No abdominal pain

indicants pointing in this direction and non against; early repletion after meals has a weight of +63 towards gastric cancer. For the lower section (Decision 2) the probability of 0.47 reached for severe (i.e. complicated oesophageal disease) is reached in two stages. Firstly the probability of oesophageal disease is calculated (not shown) and then the factors indicating complicated disease are listed. For example the short history adds 128 to the score; the absence of dysphagia and the sex of the patient are against this, but the overall score favours severe oesophageal disease. To the doctor using the system the list of symptoms are both explanatory and also educational, in the sense that the weights could be learned if desired from the printout. Contradictory symptoms (those against diagnosis) can be checked by further questioning of the patient if desired.

Secondly, the list of probabilities are given in descending order (as in Table 6) and thirdly, a simple list of all the symptoms which the patient admits to, is included (not illustrated).

INITIAL INFORMAL ASSESSMENT OF 'GLADYS'
(Glasgow dyspepsia system)

It has been noted above that the data base for the programme has been obtained using patients from the lists of the G.P.s now participating in the primary care trial. Validation of the diagnostic probabilities generated by the computer is important and is assisted by the common geographical and social background of the G.P. and hospital population.

Comparisons were undertaken between two groups of patients comprising the first 79 referred to the Health Centre and a group of 100 seen concurrently at the Southern General Hospital. These patients were looked at in detail and the spread of calculated probabilities examined. The only differences which came to light were ones which would have been expected empirically. Duodenal ulcer disease was considered more prevalent in the patients seen in General Practice. Irritable Bowel Syndrome (IBS) on the other hand was significantly more frequent a diagnosis in the hospital group. The only other comparison which showed significant variation between the groups was that a definitive (high calculated probability) gastroenterological diagnosis was more likely in a population seen by hospital G.I. service. High probabilities of a disease were therefore common in the hospital population. Low probabilities (less than 0.05) were more common than expected at Govan for 3 diagnostic categories, namely, gastric cancer, organic bowel disease and "insufficient evidence". Thus there is no indication that the questionnaire used and the statistical likelihoods obtained using hospital based data provide unexpected results when applied to a G.P. population.

CONTROLLED TRIAL

There are a large number of potential outcome measures to consider when undertaking a randomised controlled trial of "GLADYS". These include -
1. Prescribing pattern
2. Referral rate
3. Radiology rate
4. Endoscopy rate
5. Laboratory investigation
6. Attitudes to computers (patients and doctors)
7. Time off work

The method used is for the patient who presents with any symptom referrable to the G.I. tract (with the exception of rectal bleeding) and who is 14 years or older to be referred by his G.P. for a computer questionnaire to be administered. There is no attempt at any stage to dictate a specific line of management to the family doctor. Patients are randomly allocated to control or experimental groups and a full printout of the diagnostic probabilities generated by the machine is given to the referring doctor for those in the experimental group. Control patients have a simple form of acknowledgement returned to their doctor. It is at this stage that each patient must be carefully monitored to detect any significant changes in the way they are handled clinically.

It is unfortunately too early to produce results for this work but as can be seen in the above list we have been able to monitor several outcome variable which give a detailed picture of the management of dyspepsia in General Practice. All patients referred to the trial are examined and the prescribing pattern analysed over the preceding six months. There is also throughout the duration of the trial observation of the continued prescriptions used. The most recent results indicate that antacids, closely followed by H2 antagonists, are the most popular drugs used in this population and also that considerable expense is involved.

Referral rates are monitored by the secretarial pool at the Health Centre which is responsible for all letters of referral. Radiology consumption has been monitored using a computerised archive based in the X-ray Department in the Southern General Hospital. Results to date are shown in Table 8 and the cost is necessarily an

Table 8

G.I. Radiology at S.G.H. over 5 months

34 GPs

Ba. Meals	−	157 (378 per annum)
Ba. Enemas	−	45 (108 per annum)
Cholecystograms	−	14 (34 per annum)
Annual Cost	−	£21,000

approximation. Endoscopy rate is observed using a separate filing system at the local G.I. Centre. Information regarding laboratory investigations and time off work are culled directly from patient records. Computer attitudes are examined using the Stanford Opinion Scale in Medical Computing originated by Teach and Shortcliffe (1981). Patient attitudes are being explored using the Attitudes Scale developed by Lucas (1977).

Conclusions

Dyspepsia is a common problem and yet is one which gives rise to a lot of uncertainty in respect of management. The development of decision aids for the condition might reduce some of the uncertainty in managing dyspepsia. There is a voluminous literature on Computer Diagnosis (105 references in the Medical Literature per year in the late 1970's) which shows but slight signs of abating (90 references a year in the 1980's); there are very few references about dyspepsia and yet it is a common condition. The system described above appears useful. It is hoped to show, within a year, whether this type of programme can contribute in a positive sense to speeding up the institution of specific appropriate therapy, reducing the consumption of expensive and time-consuming hospital investigations and perhaps to reducing patients' time off work by reducing morbidity experienced as a result of delay before appropriate treatment is started. We think that the statistical basis of GLADYS, based as it is on the probabilistic paradigm, is sound and derived from fastidiously collected data; futhermore the nature of the output should help acceptance in the wider medical community and remind others that diagnostic aids based on statistical inference can also explain the reasons for their suggestions.

REFERENCES

Anonymous. British Medical Journal, (1978) 1, 1163-1164.

Card, W.I., Nicholson, M., Crean, G.P., Watkinson, G., Evans, C.R. and Wilson, J., (1974) International Journal of Bio-Medical Computing, 5, 175-187.

Card, W.I., and Lucas, R.W., (1981) International Journal of Man-Machine Studies, 14, 49-57.

Hannay, D.R., (1978) The Symptom Iceberg. Routledge & Kegan Paul.

Lucas, R.W., Card, W.I., Knill-Jones, R.P., Watkinson, G. and Crean, G.P. (1976) British Medical Journal, 2, 623-625.

Lucas, R.W., (1977) International Journal of Man-Machine Studies, 9, 69-86.

Spiegelhalter, D.J., and Knill-Jones, R.P., (1984) Journal of the Royal Statistical Society (A), 147, 35-77.

Teach, R.L., and Shortliffe, E.H. (1981) Computing and Biomedical Research, 14, 542-587.

21
The Health Problem and Tools for the Computer

Bent Guttorm Bentsen

Defining the health problems of a person has been a growing concern for health care during the last few years.

A definition of a health problem could be: Anything that has, or may require, health care management and has, or could significantly affect a person's physical or emotional well-being. Also included are social problems affecting health. The health problem can either be as presented by the person concerned or as defined by the professional (Sandlow et al., 1974; WONCA, 1981; Bentsen, 1976a).

Aetiology of disease and the "machine failure" of organ or organ systems have been in the centre of medical research and education for 100 years. Textbooks have concentrated on diseases often only defined by a cluster of complaints or signs of disease. The "world" has been that of the hospitals, and it seems that the rule of "the more rare, the more important" have often dominated the medical community's mind. Medical specialities have been developed and organised in hospitals, and around organs and organ systems.

At last a rethinking is taking place. There is reaction against the reductive, simplifying way of thinking, towards complexity and reality. This reductionism, represented by the laboratory with all its triumphs, has met a challenge: - the holistic way of thinking. This revolution has been going on during the last few years affecting medicine and many other disciplines. From physics and mathematics, to history research, sociology and philosophy. In medicine terms like problem identification, problem assessment, and problem-solving are now commonly accepted, and in medical research "soft" data have been accepted beside "hard" data.

The computer has to a large extent made it possible to analyse and understand the holistic, primary care paradigm. The computer has made it possible to handle complex and large data sets, - and letting these undergo advanced statistical analyses. Terms like "Bayes' theorem" (Galen and Gambino, 1975), and "probabilities" are often used. We can follow the details of a person's life through many years. We can assess these details in relation to both personal and social factors. We can learn about "normality", "well-being", "diagnosing" and "treatment". The basic concept is that every person is unique, different from all other persons.

WHY ANALYSE THE DIAGNOSTIC PROCESS?

Many reasons for analysing the diagnostic process have been presented. Three could be stressed:

- It is of importance for undergraduate teaching in medical schools. Much more of the teaching should be focused on problem-solving. This implies also problem identification and problem assessment. Statistical analyses of what is going on in primary care can teach us how this is best done.

- It is of importance for graduate and postgraduate education of primary care physicians; maybe it is of importance to all members of the medical profession. We need to know more about diagnostic strategies, therapeutic strategies, and the natural history of disease. We need to know about the predictive value of tests or anamnestic questions, or the probability of a certain disease process given a certain complaint.

- It is of importance for the identification of general medical practice or family medicine as a medical discipline of its own right.

HOW TO ANALYSE THE DIAGNOSTIC PROCESS?

Looking at the diagnostic process is just like looking at slides from the time our children were growing up. The child was a baby, then two years old, and then .... This reflects the primary physicians' "step by step method" (Bentsen, 1980a). We can observe a person at certain points of time, but we do not really know what is happening in between encounters.

Figure 1 shows a data structure for analyses of the diagnostic process (Engelsaastro, 1979). The structure is person orientated. That means that every person must have a unique identification number which functions as the main key to the data base. The data base will primarily include basic information about the person such as age and sex.

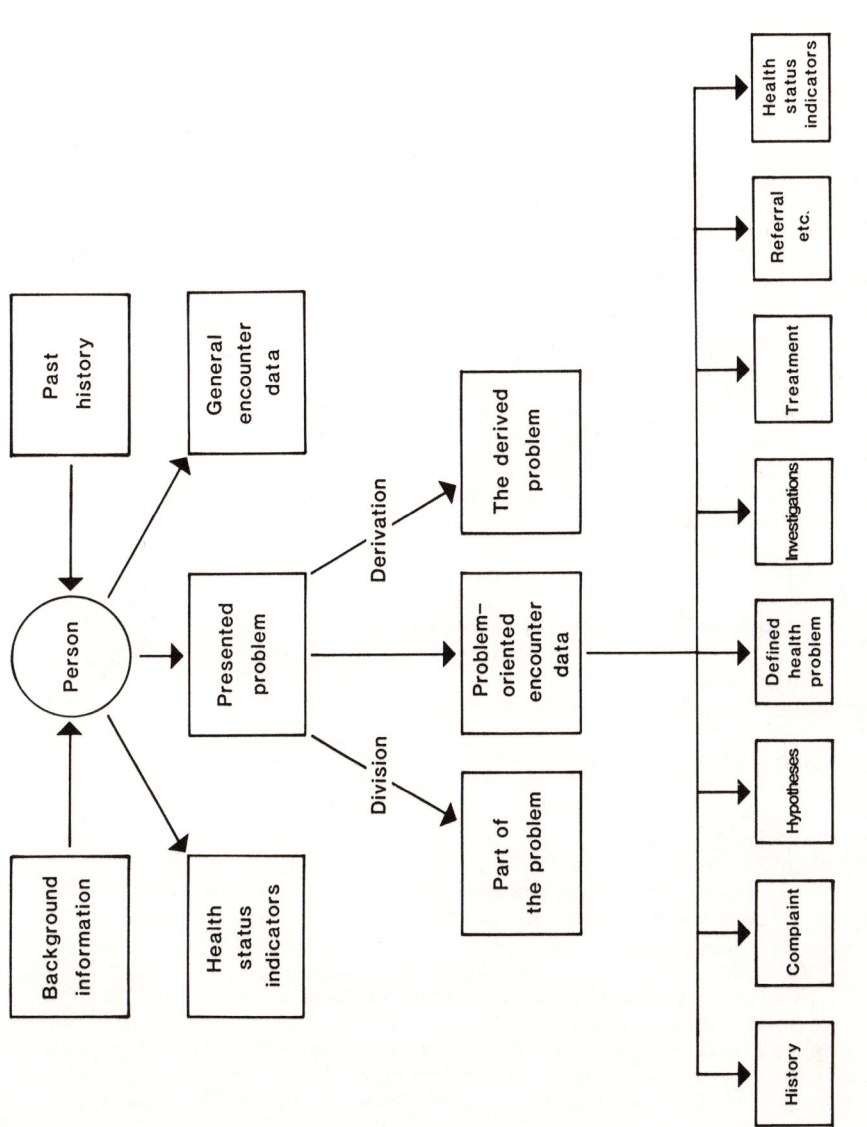

Figure 1   A Datastructure for Analyses of the Diagnostic Process

224 Decision-making in General Practice

The arrows show the logical lines to different postclasses. Some of the information about the encounter will be a general description of the contact and directly be related to the person. Other items of person-related information is the patient's background i.e. family or living conditions, past experiences of disease, and the health status of the person.

However, a patient can have several separate, independent health problems at the same time either to be diagnosed or under treatment (Bentsen, 1976b). The data-structure makes it possible to split one health problem into several different parts, and also to "redefine" several problems to one. It also allows an unlimited number of encounters concerning a health problem. During every contact the status of the problem is recorded: if it is new, under analysis or treatment, or if it is finished. Clinical information, investigation and test results, treatment, information about referral to other health care professional, and the health status of the patient will be recorded.

DIFFICULTIES IN THE RECORDING OF DATA

Two problems concerning the recording of data will be commented on:

a) the presented problems' relation to the final defined problems,

and

b) the problem of multidiagnostics.

The defined health problems of professionals may often seem to be far away from the primarily presented ones.

Figure 2 shows a situation where a patient is presenting a health problem. The professional wishes to split this into two separate problems which we may call (P1a) and (P1b). These are then recorded as "new problems" (P2 and P3), but behind is added "Derived from problem P1" or DFP1.

Figure 3 shows the opposite situation. The physician may have believed he is presented several different, independent problems, but that these really were parts of one common problem. To the "New problem" should therefore be added DFP1, DFP2 and DFP3.

Figure 4 shows a situation which is a combination of Figure 2 and Figure 3. This example of a problem-structure shows that the patient originally presented two problems. The physician decided that these, in fact, represented four different problems. Finally, this ended up as

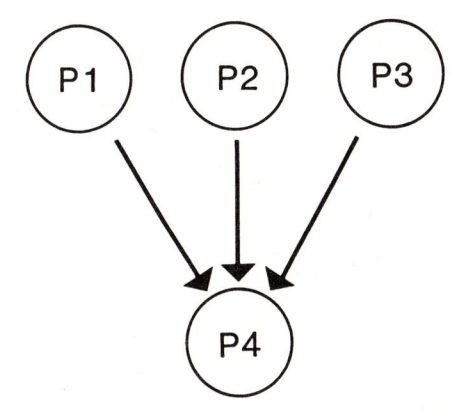

The Health Problem and Tools for the Computer 225

**THREE PROBLEMS PRESENTED
REPRESENTING
ONLY ONE PROBLEM.**

Figure 2

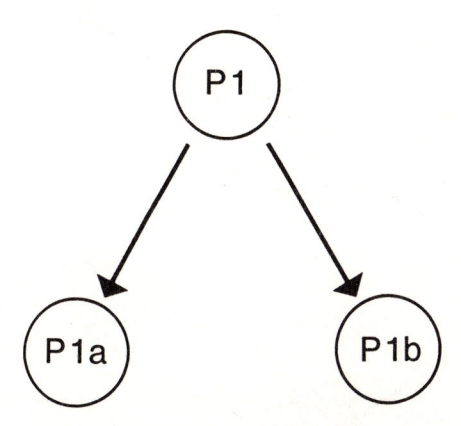

**ONE PROBLEM PRESENTED,
REPRESENTING
TWO DIFFERENT PROBLEMS.**

Figure 3

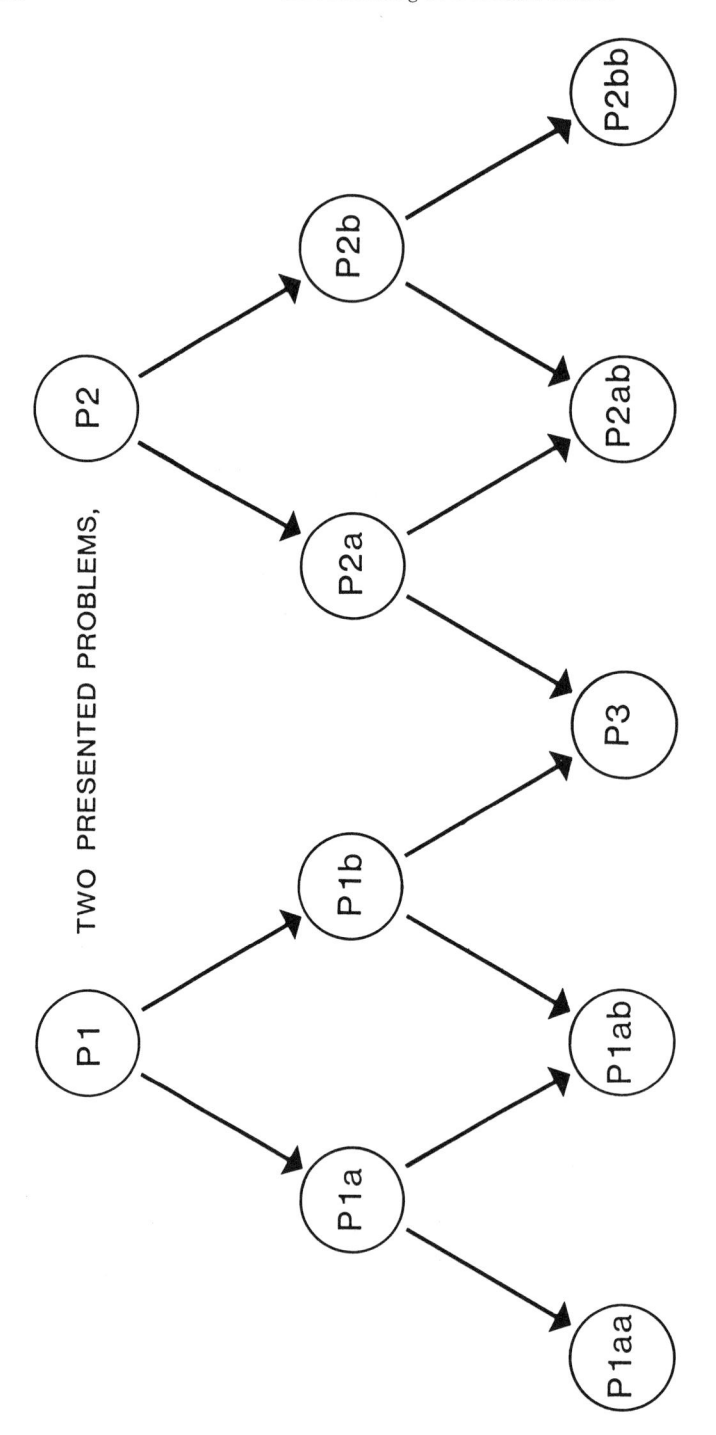

REPRESENTING FIVE DIFFERENT PROBLEMS, TWO PRESENTED PROBLEMS

Figure 4

five different problems; two were redefined to represent one, and the others were again split up. The primary physician is concerned with a complex world. However, the marking of the single problem on its way to the final, defined one, makes it possible to keep track. It is just like using tracer elements.

The diagnostic process is very complex (McWhinney, 1972; Bentsen, 1980b). The fact that so often more than one health problem is presented by the patient during the same encounter, up to 8-10, and with an average of 2.5, faces the primary physician with a challenge (Bentsen, 1976b). The study referred to comprised 57 residents at family medicine graduate training programme, and three pairs of independent, experienced general practitioners as observers.

The "generalist" has the responsibility of meeting the needs of people with problems. That concerns all aspects of a human being, - physical, emotional and social problems (Bentsen, 1970). It is regrettable that we still search for a vocabulary being fully able to reflect the realities of life (Dixon, 1983).

THE BASE FOR A DATA SYSTEM

However, we are on the way. During the last few years The Classification Committee of WONCA (The World Organisation of National Colleges, Academics and Academic Associations of General Practitioner/Family Physicians) has done a good job. Since 1972 the committee has worked on classifications and definitions of terms, developing further the work of others, (for example the Royal College of General Practitioners). Close co-operation has also been established between WHO and WONCA.

Some major instruments for making analysis of the diagnostic process possible can be presented. At least three requirements must be met for any such instrument:

- It must undergo a feasibility study in the daily practice of physicians in many different countries.

- It must be generally accepted by representative organisations, and by professionals using the classifications.

- It must be simple and operational.

These requirements have been met in the work of the Classification Committee of WONCA. In the following sections the International Glossary and the work of Classifications will be described.

AN INTERNATIONAL GLOSSARY FOR PRIMARY CARE

Precise definitions of terms which describe the process of primary care are essential to the collection of primary health care data. Whenever possible, these definitions should be uniform and unambiguous. Research workers who wish to collaborate with or interpret work of colleagues from other countries can benefit from a standard glossary of commonly used health terms. In response to these needs the Classification Committee of WONCA has defined an international glossary.

Consensus on definitions was reached by the Committee with consultation from general practice/family medicine organisations and individuals. Existing primary care glossaries from several countries and the World Health Organisation were also consulted.

The definitions provided are intended as guidelines, rather than absolute dicta, for primary care providers and researchers who desire comparability. New knowledge, drifts in use of language with time, and new processes will inevitably require revision of definitions and the addition of new terms. A comprehensive dictionary is not intended, rather the inclusion of most commonly used terms.

The Glossary comprises nine chapters:

1. General
2. Provider Descriptors
3. Practice Descriptors
4. Patient Descriptors
5. Population Descriptors
6. Morbidity Descriptors
7. Encounter Descriptors
8. Service Descriptors
9. Standard Reporting

A few examples are given here:

I. General

A. Health - A state of optimal physical, mental and social well-being, and not merely the absence of disease or infirmity (modified World Health Organisation definition).

B. Health Care - Assessment, health maintenance, therapy, education, promotion of health, prevention of illness, and related activities (provided by qualified professionals) to improve or maintain health status.

C. Health care system - The organisational structure through which health care is provided.

VII. Encounter Descriptions

A. Encounter - Any professional interchange between a patient and one or more members of a health care team. One or more problems or diagnoses may be identified at each encounter. Analyses of encounter data should distinguish encounters from problems.

1. Direct Encounter (Face-to-Face Meeting) - An encounter in which there is a face-to-face meeting of a patient and professional.

2. Indirect Encounter - An encounter in which there is no physical or face-to-face meeting between the patient and the professional.

The different types of direct or indirect encounters are then specified. The term encounter was chosen because "visit" or "consultation" have different interpretations in different countries.

THE REASON FOR ENCOUNTER CLASSIFICATION FOR USE IN PRIMARY CARE

The Reason for Encounter Classification (ICPC - The International Classification of Primary Care) (Lamberts, 1982; WHO, 1980) is designed by a WHO Working Party to classify the reasons why patients seek care at the primary level. A patient makes contact with the health care system by requesting services from a primary care provider. The provider first identifies the stated purpose or reason for contact, then as the information base increases, defines the problem and carries out the appropriate actions required to provide health care. By definition, the reason for encounter is the agreed statement of the reason(s) why a person enters the health care system. The terms written down by the provider should be recognised by the patient as an acceptable description of this reason while it also represents the starting point for action by the provider.

DESCRIPTION OF THE ICPC

The ICPC is designed along two axes: Chapters and Components (Figure 5). Thirteen chapters are titled by body systems, in addition there are three titled "General", "Psychological", and "Social".

There are no chapters on infectious diseases, neoplasms, injuries and congenital anomalies like those in the ICD-9, while these conditions are represented in the Diagnosis/Disease component of the chapters. Each chapter carried an alpha-code which is the first character of the basic 3 character alphanumeric code. Each chapter is subdivided into seven "components" (Figure 5).

These components are consistent throughout all chapters. The components carry a 2-digit numeric code which follows the alpha.

RELATION OF ICPC TO EXISTING CLASSIFICATION

ICPC was influenced by existing major classifications. ICD-9 forms the basis for component 7, the Disease/Diagnosis component; the International Classification of Health Problems in Primary Care (WONCA, 1983) - ICHPPC-2 or ICD-9 General Medicine - practically reflects this component.

The Symptoms/Complaints component drew from the existing National Ambulatory Medical Care Survey/Reason for Visit Classification (NAMCS/RFV) (National Centre for Health Statistics, 1979; National Ambulatory Medical Services, 1981).

Components 2 and 3, Diagnostic, Screening, Preventive, and Treatment and Medication, interface with the ICD-9 Procedures in Medicine (WHO, 1978) and the North American Primary Care Research Group (NAPCRG-1) Process Code for Primary Care (NAPCRG, 1981; Tindall et al. 1981). The WHO-sponsored Triaxial Classification (WHO, 1979) focuses on the classification of psychological, social and organic problems.

The axes covering psychological and social problems have been replicated in the ICPC as chapters P and Z respectively. Thus, the scheme of the ICPC emerges as a possible core classification for the ICD-10 family of classifications (Kupka, 1978).

AN ICPC FEASIBILITY STUDY

The ICPC classification is currently undergoing a feasibility study. General practitioners and nurses in 10 different countries all over the world have been recording the reasons which patients expressed as to why contact was established.

All of the comments from the participants will now be assessed by the WHO Working Party on Primary Health Care Classifications. In late 1984 a final version of ICPC will be published.

The Reason for Encounter Classification provides a new paradigm for applying labels to the several stages of primary care.

The nomenclature of ICPC can be used both as a clarification of the reason for encounter and as the diagnosis (Relation with ICHPPC-2). Apart from this ICPC allows us to classify the process of care (components 2-6). This is important for a problem oriented approach to health care.

The nomenclature of ICPC with one index and one set of synonyms thus serves to classify three of the four SOAP elements: Subjective, Assessment, Plan. Objective findings cannot be classified with the nomenclature of ICPC.

Figure 5 shows the rubrics of Component 2 - 6 of all Chapters and Components 1 and 7 of the first Chapter (A) as they are included in

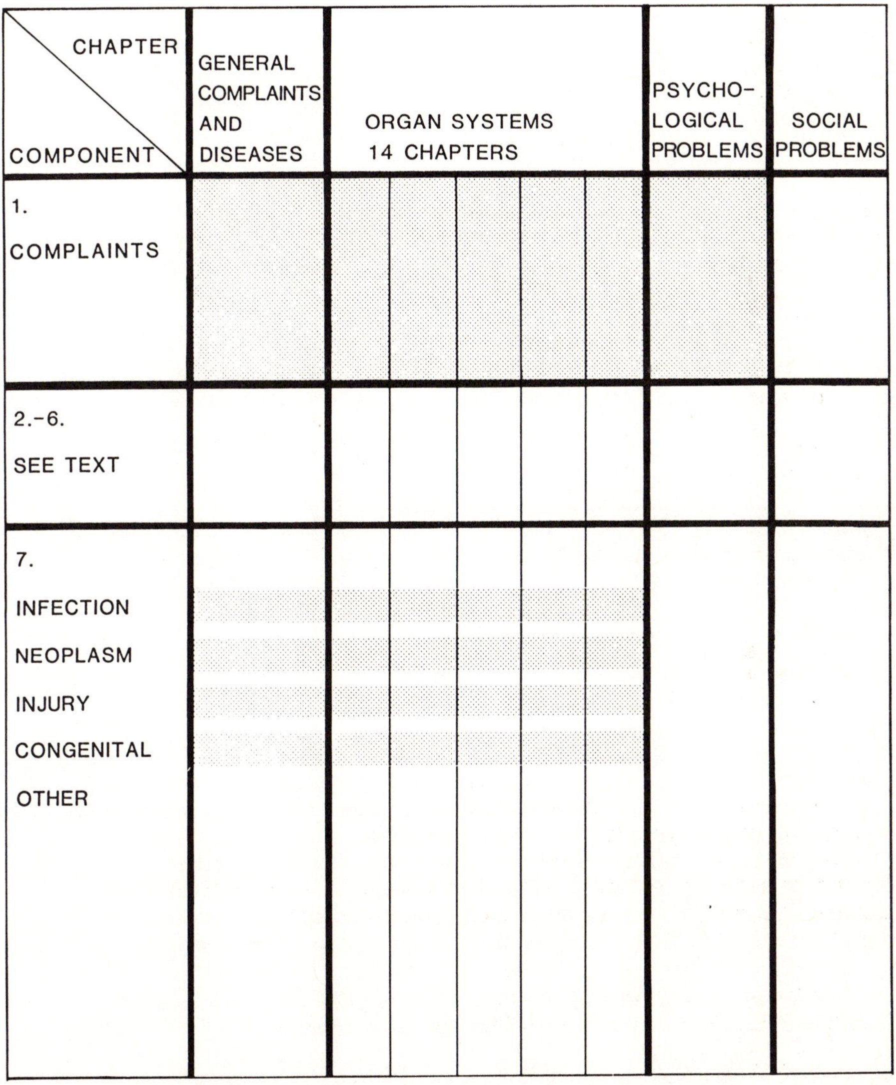

CHAPTER \ COMPONENT	GENERAL COMPLAINTS AND DISEASES	ORGAN SYSTEMS 14 CHAPTERS			PSYCHO- LOGICAL PROBLEMS	SOCIAL PROBLEMS
1. COMPLAINTS						
2.-6. SEE TEXT						
7. INFECTION NEOPLASM INJURY CONGENITAL OTHER						

Figure 5 Format of International Classification of Primary Care (ICPC). The Chapters and Components Form Two Axes

the field of trial version of ICPC. This example illustrates the format of the new classification system and its mnemonic advantages when used in everyday pratice.

ICHPPC-2-DEFINED

After several years of successful and ever-increasing use of ICHPPC (International Classification of Health Problems in Primary Care), a new edition of this Classification was edited in 1981 (WONCA, 1981).

The ICHPPC-1 was derived from the International Classification of Diseases, Eighth Revision (ICD-8), which was subsequently revised as ICHPPC-2, in order to make it compatible with the then new revision of ICD-9. This new publication, as its predecessor, represents an adaptation for general practice and, in addition to diagnoses, consists mainly of rubrics related to other problems encountered in primary health care. The new major feature is the fact that an attempt has been made to define by selection criteria the majority of terms used in the Classification, and therefore ICHPPC-2 becomes ICHPPC-2 Defined. It is expected that this modification will remarkably increase its usefulness by introducing the standarised inclusion criteria and terms in addition to the Classification.

These criteria and terms are not necessarily the same as those used or being developed by the World Health Organisation. This also applies to the International glossary for general practice/family practice. However, the World Health Organisation has welcomed this important effort to enhance communication with and among general practitioners and family physicians.

There is no difference between the numbering system and content of rubrics as compared to ICHPPC-2.

PURPOSE

The spectrum of ICHPPC includes the content of primary care: the health problems in people who feel ill, as well as those who consider themselves to be healthy but seek expert primary medical care evaluation and advice. ICHPPC is so devised that valid and reliable statistical comparisons may be made between morbidity or workload reports from front-line medical practices anywhere in the world.

The following features of ICHPPC bore heavily on its design, its development, and the organisation for its maintenance.

a) ICHPPC represents a consensus on the content of primary care derived from the wide practical experience of many different general practitioners/family physicians from several countries.

b) Its broad-based input facilitates its adaption to changes in concepts of health and disease, and to new developments in primary health care delivery.

c) The "optional hierarchy" principle enables ICHPPC to accomodate recording problems of local importance and those of special interest to recorders, without threatening comparability.

d) The full spectrum of first contact medicine is covered: ICHPPC can be used comfortably by health workers of various disciplines, in any setting from single-handed rural practice to the emergency department of a university hospital.

e) The brevity and simplicity of the list makes its use as effective for a secretary with pencil and paper as for a well-staffed medical records department with computer facilities.

f) While specifically directed towards the needs of primary care, ICHPPC-2, by virtue of its close alignment with the International Classification of Diseases - Ninth Revision (ICD-9), permits comparisons with work from other fields of medicine.

A PROCESS CODE FOR PRIMARY CARE

The World Health Organisation has worked out an International Classification of Procedures in Medicine (WHO, 1978). However, this is not adaptable for use in primary care. Also many other classifications of procedure have been developed to meet the needs of particular providers or third party payer organisations. Many of these systems have a relationship to each other, but because of the lack of a common organising body, sufficient changes took place in the development of each of these that effective comparisons are seldom possible. Their comprehensiveness and unwieldy construction and arrangement made them ill-suited for the purposes of primary care.

NAPCRG (North America Primary Care Research Group) therefore found it necessary to work out a general accepted classification for diagnostic and therapeutic procedures for North America (NAPCRG, 1981). This classification has now been field tested worldwide by the Classification Committee of WONCA. At the end of 1984 a final version of a WONCA Classification for Procedures will be published.

This classification is also hierarchical, using a three- or four-digit code. The 2 digit code offers a relatively non-specific classification, and will probably be too broad for most users. However, it should prove useful in the comparative studies where great specificity is not desirable. The 3 digit code may prove the most useful for many users.

The 4 digit code was designed to follow the ICHPPC-2 format as much as possible. Bear in mind, however, that ICHPPC-2 is not a completely hierarchical code and cannot be collapsed into a 3 and 2 digit code, as the NAPCRG Process Code can.

Many of the NAPCRG 4 digit code numbers are identical with ICHPPC-2 code numbers. Providers integrating both sets of code numbers into one system may want to provide a designator or other mechanism to separate the two coding systems.

The Process Code is intended as a companion coding system to ICHPPC-2, and as such, it is hoped that it will be a major step towards the long term goal expressed in ICHPPC-2, i.e. "to provide agreement on classification for ... the process - what the provider does for the patient". Although labelled as "process", which implies that the code is restricted to management, there is a section devoted to "Site and Duration of Service". In conjunction with ICPC and ICHPPC-2, the NAPCRG Process Code is intended to provide a simple classification system for all of the items normally monitored in primary health care, other than direct outcome items such as laboratory results. The three coding systems used together should afford the user a method of recording what problems health providers see, where the encounter occurred, the length of time involved, the management of the problem, and the disposition of the patient.

HEALTH STATUS INDICATORS

Figure 1 displays many "post classes" in a data system. This presentation has shown how box after box in the data structure has been filled in with internationally accepted definitions and classifications. However, there are still areas left: i.e. the open boxes for Health Status Indicators. The Classification Committee of WONCA and WHO has now started working on Health Status Indicators.

These will probably comprise the following (Kupka, 1978, Bentsen, 1970, 1983)

- Person characteristics:

  Socio-economic level, personal occupation, degree of employment, family educational level.

- Disability:

  Activities of daily living, social functioning, dependency, pain/discomfort, fitness.

- Morbidity:

  Characteristics of the Health problem, duration, effect on functional capacity.

- Vulnerability:

    Prognosis of the health problem, occupational prognosis, stress resources, personality traits, health attitudes, quality of nutrition, quality of housing.

- Well-being:

    Family cohesion, work satisfaction, use of free time, time living in the area, involvement in community.

- Perception of health

Over the last few years much has been achieved through international cooperation. The challenge of defining Health Status Indicators will keep many people busy for years ahead.

DOES THE DATA SYSTEM WORK

The system referred to in Figure 1 has been tested (Engelsaastro, 1979), having originally been designed for a research practice in the Aafjord district, Norway. If the resources are sufficient, the data structure presented can routinely be used, or it can be used to analyse specific questions or hypotheses. These may comprise i.e. the natural history of disease, guidelines for diagnosing or treatment, the predictive value of tests, the probability of a certain disease given a certain symptom, and even help us to define "normality" or "well-being". The system can also take account of the wide area of psycho-social factors in a person's life.

REFERENCES

Bentsen, B.G., (1970). Illness and general practice. A survey of medical care of an inland population in south-east of Norway. University Press, Oslo-Bergen-Tromso. p.192.

Bentsen, B.G., (1976a). Classifying of health problems in primary medical care. Journal of Royal College of General Practitioners (Occasional Paper 1), pp.1-5.

Bentsen, B.G., (1976b). The accuracy of recording patient problems in family practice. Journal of Medical Education. 51, 311-316.

Bentsen, B.G., (1980a). Working techniques. In: Primary Care. (ed. J.Fry) William Heinemanns Medical Books Ltd., London; 340-344.

Bentsen, B.G., (1980b). The diagnostic process in primary medical care. In: Primary Care. (ed. J.Fry). William Heinemanns Medical Books Ltd., London; 328-339.

Bentsen, B.G., (1983). Can Health be measured? Conference Proceedings. Tenth WONCA World Conference on Family Medicine. Singapore; 105-109.

Dixon, A.S., (1983). Family Medicine - at a loss for words. Journal of the Royal College of General Practitioners. 33, 358-363.

Engelsaastro, E., (1979). Aafjordprosjektet. Dataregistreringsopplegg og datastruktur. Arbeidsrapport NIS. (The Aafjord Project. A Plan for recording data and its structure.)

Galen, R.S., and Gambino, S.R., (1975). Beyond normality. The predictive value and efficiency of medical diagnoses. John Wiley and Sons, New York.

Kupka, K., (1978). International classification of diseases: Ninth Revision. WHO Chronicle, 32, 219-225.

Lamberts, H., (1982). Redenen om naar de huisarts te gaan. Huisarts en Wetenschap, 25, 301-310.

McWhinney, I., (1972). Problem-solving and decision-making in primary medical practice. Proceedings Royal Society of Medicine, 65, 34-38.

National Ambulatory Medical Services, U.S., 1977-78. (1981). Patients' reasons for visiting physicians. Data from the National Health Survey, Hyattsville, Maryland, Series 13, No. 56, DHHS Publications; 82, 1717.

National Center for Health Statistics. (1979). A reason for visit classification for ambulatory care. U.S. Public Health Service, DHEW Publication, Hyattsville, Maryland, 79, 1352.

North American Primary Care Research Group. (1981). A process for primary care (NAPCRG-1). International field trial version. Richmond, Virginia.

Sandlow, L., Hammet, H., and Bashook, P.G., (1974). Illinois committee for problem oriented medical records. Michael Reese Medical Center, Chicago, 41.

Tindall, H.L., et. al., (1981). The NAPCRG process classification for primary care. Family Practitioner, 12, 199-200.

West, R., (1983). Health status survey. Auckland (in progress).

World Health Organization. (1978). International classification of procedures in medicine. Geneva.

World Health Organization. (1979). Psychosocial factors affecting health assessment classification and utilization workshop. Report of the World Health Organization on the Conference at Bellagio, Italy, November 6-10, 1979. Paper No. MNH/80. WHO, Geneva.

World Health Organization. (1980). Working Party. report to develop a classification of the 'Reasons for encounter with primary health care services'. Working Party report to the ICD Unit of World Health Organization, Geneva, Switzerland.

WONCA. (1981). Classification Committee of WONCA. An International glossary for primary care. Family Practitioner. 13, 673-681.

WONCA. (1983). Classification Committee of WONCA. ICHPPC-2 - Defined. (International classification of health problems in primary care). University Press, Oxford.

22
The Paper Patient — A Device for Investigation into General Practice

J. Ridderikhoff

Like most things in the medical world, the theoretical background of general practice is still in statu nascendi. Economic problems in health care, social criticism and the birth and development of medical decision-making all question medicine as it stands. This criticism implies that we are on the wrong track when we try to understand decision behaviour with the aid of normative models (expected utility, Bayesian and a few other theories). Instead we should concentrate on what people actually do and develop descriptive models to account for decision processes.

Deepening our insight into the medical process is the task of the individual doctor, in our case the general practitioner. The question is: What to study and how to study it? In my opinion, the essence of the general practitioner's functioning lies in his contacts with the patient.

The doctor has to make decisions in an uncertain problem situation which involves two systems - his own and that of the patient. From this, the main problem arises because studying the functioning of the general practitioner means observing these two systems which, at the same time, influence each other in a special implicit way. It is like focussing on a certain point on a turning wheel while sitting on another wheel rotating in the opposite direction. One observes flashes, only partly recognisable.

In order to investigate the problem-solving process between the patient and the doctor, one has to freeze one of the two systems. Studying the doctor automatically includes a "fixed" patient (and vice versa). A "fixed" patient is a simulated patient. Generally speaking, there are three possibilities for patient simulation:

- the cueing problem: suggesting questions, options or categories to the testee that otherwise might not have crossed his mind

- the question of validity; this will be discussed below

Written Simulation Informally Structured

This category contains a number of variants from the oldest simulation technique format, that of Rimoldi, as based on the tab-item technique (Glaser et al., 1952).

The case history of the patient is written on a series of cards. Each card represents a patient attribute. The "patient" is interrogated by picking cards. On the front of the cards preformulated questions are shown. The question that most nearly conforms with one's own question is picked up. The clinical information relevant to this question is printed on the reverse of each card. A number of variants to this format have been developed over the past fifteen years. Representatives of this method are: Rimoldi's 'Technique for Problem-Solving' (Rimoldi, 1961), 'Portable Patient Problem Pack' (P4) and its extension, P3 (Tamblyn & Barrow, 1978a, 1978b), 'Diagnostic Management Problem' (DMP) (Helfer & Slater, 1971), 'Minisim Mode' (Dombal et al., 1971) and 'Interactive Patient Simulation' (IPS) (Gerritsma & Smal, 1982).

The advantages are:

- challenges problem-solving skills

- allows the student or physician to follow his own reasoning path-ways

- good scoring possibilities of the separate data

The disadvantages are:

- extensive cueing

- ostensible freedom of pathways (there is no other information available than that provided for in the original medical record or composed by the expert-group)

- impossibility of scoring individual ways of reasoning.

Actor/Operator Simulations (Using the Spoken Word)

This category can be divided into two sub-classes:

Actor Simulation   An actor, usually an interested layman, trained to simulate patients, is provided with a detailed synopsis of the personal and medical history part of a patient problem.

The advantages are:

- challenging problem-solving abilities

- allows the testee/trainee to follow his own pathways

- high validity (high fidelity) to clinical situations

The disadvantages are:

- high costs

- limitation in use of the actor, not only on account of availability but for shifts in role-content

- more difficult scoring dependent on expert judgements

- limited range of measurement of clinical competence (neglecting the data processing from physical examination, laboratory tests, etc.)

Verbal Mode   The patient's case history is recorded in a pre-structured system (cards, books). The user asks questions verbally to an operator as though he, the operator, is the patient. The answers are provided through the operator from the 'written' system.

Advantages of this mixed (written and spoken word) system are:

- challenges problem-solving abilities

- allows the testee/trainee to follow his own cognitive workup

Disadvantages are:

- the use of a competent, available operator

- extensive data gathering

- setting up of an extensive data-base for reliable scoring-indicators

(a) "Actors" simulating patients.

(b) Written simulations (with or without the intervention of a simulator).

(c) Computerized simulations (with screen display and data storage).

Each of these techniques has its advantages and disadvantages which will be discussed in detail later on. Most techniques are more concerned with the study of mental products (e.g. examinations, accurate diagnosis) than with the study of the processes leading to the solution of a problem. They are not only goal-directed but also cover few medical fields.

For our purpose - studying the problem-solving processes of general practitioners - we need a device that suits the purpose of storing a large number of data. These data must be highly flexible, must cover a broad area of symptoms and signs and should be easy to prodnce and manage. They must also fulfil the requirements of realism and above all they must be cost-effective.

ADVANTAGES AND DISADVANTAGES OF PATIENT SIMULATION FORMATS

Written Simulations Formally Structured

Essentially, paper patients are case histories narrated in the time sequence of the real patient. For this type of paper patient, the case history is formally structured by its composers, usually a group of clinical experts. These simulations range from 'The Modified Essay Question' (Charvat et al., 1968; Kleinmuntz, 1963), a case history divided into several parts with a number of (multiple choice) questions at every interruption, to the 'Patient Management Problem' (PMP) (McCarthy & Gonella, 1967) and its many variants. The practical eliciting of the answers and the easy scoring system made this kind of simulation a popular and frequently applied instrument. The advantages are:

- good challenge to problem-solving skills

- easy and immediate responses to good and bad moves

- easy and objective scoring system

The disadvantages are:

- the student (or physician) is not free to follow his own cognitive pathways

The Paper Patient — A Device for Investigation into General Practice

Computerised simulations (CASE = Computer-Assisted Simulation Equipment) are omitted in this concise overview. Not only is there no essential difference between written or displayed information, but the clinical content for most computer-assisted instructions (Harless et al., 1971; Taylor, 1972) for the clinical content are based on one of the former categories.

The Case of Validity

All simulations are based on the assumption that the workup of the simulated clinical problem is comparable to the actions physicians have taken by solving a similar clinical problem with an actual patient. The validity of the simulation is the comparison between the registered values of the test and the values in the real world. The ideal validity would be:

$$\text{Registered Values} = \text{Actual Values}$$

One of the basic problems is that a number of qualities of the actual process are unknown or at least cannot be quantified by reliable instruments. Therefore, a formal judgment about the validity of an intrument is not directly possible. A number of procedures have been originated that indirectly give us indications about the validity of any measurement. These procedures are:

1. Content- or Face-Validity: Gives evidence about the nature of the intellectual process which the testee must go through in order to respond to a simulation. The content, the diagnostic process, in the natural setting must be (almost) the same as the one in simulation.

2. Construct Validity (Cronbach & Meehl, 1955): Gives evidence about the extent to which the performance of different groups on these exercises corresponds with reasonable hypotheses about the degree to which such groups differ. In other words, the theory, the concept on which the construction of the model is based is tested against empirical values in the real setting.

3. Concurrent Validity: Gives evidence about the relationship between scores on these exercises and the performance in other tests or settings. The comparison between the measurements of two (or more) instruments about the same elements gives an indication of the validity of one of these instruments (McGuire, 1976; Segers, 1977).

4. Predictive Validity (Groot, 1961): Gives evidence about a variable that can predict a desired criterion. The correlation between the forecasting variable and the criterion is an operational definition for predictive validity.

What we really want to know is whether present performance is indicative of future performance in a similar setting. It is assumed that the correlation between student and expert performance (the criterion) will predict skilful problem-solving behaviour of the student in the future; thus far this statement has not been verified.

Simulation in Research

The goal determines the means. In education, the objective in using a paper patient is quite obvious, but in research there are a large number of goals. Each of them requires special measurement and, therefore, a special instrument.

If the investigator has chosen simulation as an intermediary between his theory and the real world, he has to see to it that the indicators of the instrument meet the variables of the theory.

The comparison of the different kinds of simulations used in studies of physicians and their practice presents the observer with several problems. The complexity of this subject forces investigators to make a selection of aspects or to choose some type of strategy. These strategies can roughly be divided into:

a) an empirically based strategy, which tries to understand who the doctor is, what he is doing, how he functions and what his effectiveness is,

and

b) an operational research strategy, where the aim is to build or to rebuild strategies according to which the medical process, the diagnostic as well as the therapeutic part, can be shaped or reshaped into an easy manageable structure. This group does not make use of simulations for research purposes.

Surprisingly little empirical research has so far been done on these professional activities. Although there is a growing interest in this field, a number of methodological limitations (already mentioned) seems to inhibit further investigations.

Uberla (1980) notes some other problems such as:

- the difficulties inherent in the formulation of feasible tasks. Substantial segments of professional medical action have never been approached in a way amenable to an empirical investigation. The process itself is inadequately formulated.

- the high level of inconstancy and variability. Diseases change the unstable equilibrium of the body functions. The equilibrium states change every time the organism tries to regulate itself. Variability from one patient to another is a still larger problem.

- the rarity of events. This rarity of specific phenomena is coupled with the huge variability inherent in medicine. Therefore, rare events can only be grasped by observing large numbers of cases, which represent another barrier to the feasibility of empirical studies.

- the incalculable totality of the phenomena involved. Dismembering of medical actions does not mean an understanding of the totality of the composing elements.

- causal relationships are very difficult to comprehend and to prove in complex systems.

- the inadequacy of theoretical models represents a serious limitation, as mentioned below.

- the lack of validated instruments for the collection of data relevant to medical dialogues and interviews, decision-making strategies, therapeutic procedures or management plans. Neither are we able to outline the utility of the outcome of medical processes.

Empirically based studies can roughly be divided into two categories:

- Studies based on reasoning processes in medical problem-solving, or, more generally speaking, medical decision analysis.

- Studies about some aspects of the physician's procedures.

The former group studies clinical decision-making in order to understand and/or imitate this type of human thinking process. The importance of these studies for medical education and the improvement of performance and productivity of the medical actions is quite obvious.

The latter group tries to analyse a number of aspects inherent to the decision-making behaviour of physicians. It focuses, for instance, on aspects such as duration of visits, number of questions, referrals, postgraduate education, choice of drugs. In a number of studies, comparisons have been made between physicians of different specialties.

Limitations of Patient Simulations

Simulations of patients have certain limitations. The inconstancy and the high variability of physicians' questions and patients' replies makes the content of the medical encounter highly unpredictable. Therefore the construction of a valid and reliable simulation instrument is a problematic work. Far more than simulation in medical education, where structures are kept within a more or less narrow framework, this type of simulation has to account for the unlimited and uninhibited boundaries of medical actions.

Limitations of Actors

It is widely assumed that actor presentation of a patient scenario is the most valid and "real" type of simulation. Whether this assumption is true remains to be seen. The actor can play his role without deviation only for a limited number of times. There are more problems concerning actor simulation such as:

- limited content: the more facts the actor has to remember, the more liable he is to confusion and to forgetting;

- restraints to the construction: the more complicated the patient scenario, the more mistakes can be made.

- restrictions of mode: in general, actors are not able to simulate the elements of physical examination or to be the data base for their biochemical or x-ray properties.

- high cost: several actors may have to be used to fulfil the demands of more extended projects.

Limitations of Paper Patients

Several limitations of paper patient simulations will be illustrated on the basis of a number of investigations:

1. Smith and McWhinney (1975) confronted nine general practitioners and nine consulting internists with three "simple and undefined patients". The project used a small number of measures:

- the frequency with which individual questions were asked

- the number of questions asked

- the number of laboratory and X-ray investigations.

A research assistant played all three patients, including medical history, physical examination and laboratory findings. Unfortunately, a number of details about the simulation were not reported, such as the number of "patient facts", the number of unanswered or negatively answered questions, the data source, the structuring and storing of the data, number of items per patient, the relevance of answered and unanswered questions, the profession of the research assistant, and his instructions.

2. Elstein, Shulman and Sprafka (1978) used three types of simulation: actor-simulation (high fidelity), written simulation (low fidelity) and fixed-order problems. The latter can be placed under the heading of "game simulation" and will not be discussed.

Three patient scenarios were prepared for the high fidelity simulation. The subject matters were well-circumscribed disease-entities from hematology, gastroenterology and neurology. In this latter case, the actress simulated, in addition to the medical history, the physical signs as well (sensory and motor losses). Laboratory and X-ray tests were provided on standard forms. The testees were instructed that they were free to elicit whatever data were felt to be necessary and in whatever order was appropriate. The procedure was interrupted for moments of "thinking aloud". How far this "thinking aloud" (a quite unnatural behaviour for the physician) disturbed the sphere of reality is not reported. Elstein et al. state that most physicians reported that the simulations were convincing and provided a satisfactory approximation of the atmosphere of a real case.

The "thinking aloud" procedure was planned in so-called natural breaks, usually between history and physical examination, and between this latter and prior to ordering laboratory tests. That means a strict division of various parts of the diagnostic process. The extent to which this sequence is natural is not addressed in the study.

The actors (with the exception of the actress) left the "consulting room" after completing the medical history. No latitude was given to re-enter the medical history in other parts of the workup. Some clinicians made remarks about this separation, as it would not be maintained in their usual method. The lack of time constraints was mentioned as being an artificial circumstance. The consultation was videotaped during the whole session. The notion that, after a short time, physicians are unaware of the cameras is affirmed by several investigators. After the workup of the three patients, the videotape was replayed to the physician urging him to think aloud and explain his thoughts and moves. This procedure is called after Kagan (1973) the "stimulated recall". How far this kind of introspection is valid for the elucidating of the ways of reasoning is still a matter of debate.

We can see the dilemma of simulation with this type of research. For the objective of their research, eliciting the medical problem-solving process, Elstein and co-workers had to imitate the real processes in a situation as free as possible, yet were forced to structure their model because of the limitations of the actors. Trying to catch the process by observation, they had to rely on disrupting and unnatural procedure (to the physician) of "thinking aloud" and introspection. Aware of the imperfection of the simulation, they were bound by the available possibilities.

The written (low fidelity) simulations were somewhat modified patient management problems by Elstein and co-workers. Fifteen out of the original group of twenty-four clinicians participated in this simulation session. They solved four patient management problems, each consisting of various sections. The entering of a section made all options visible to the testee and, therefore, could have served as cues for choices. Modifications on the PMPs were introduced with regard to the recording of the sequence of chosen options and to registration of hypotheses at the end of each section. The former instruction was found to be an unreasonable constraint on normal behaviour and the testees neglected it. The latter item was introduced after the results of the high fidelity study with regard to the early hypothesis generation became aware to the investigators. How far this introduction has methodological implications is beyond the scope of this paper.

The problems and limitations of the PMP format were only partly elicited in the study. A supplementary problem was that only about sixty percent of the original participants joined the second round. Because of this adventitious circumstance, conclusions from this part of the research project can hardly be drawn. Investigators have to be aware of this incidental restriction. Several methodological questions about this research remain to be answered (see also McGaghie (1980). Related to the inspiring theoretical concept, this study can be marked as one of the most ambitious of the last ten years.

Gerritsma and Smal (1982) recently completed a comparison of the working methods of general practitioners and consulting internists. It can be viewed as an extension of the study by Smith and McWhinney (1975). Gerritsma and Smal used a new simulation technique, the 'Interactive Patient Simulation' (IPS). It is based on the 'Diagnostic Management Problem' (DMP) model of Helfer and Slater (1971), which is a variant of the Rimoldi technique. The system consists of about 1600 options arranged under about one hundred headings. Apart from the personal and social information, the headings are named after the organ systems (respiratory, circulation, digestive tract, etc.) as well as the (larger) anatomical parts of the body (head, thorax, abdomen, etc.). Options belonging to more than one category are repeated. There are four headings designed for systematic (algorithmic) questioning. The number of "patients" is limited to two, but this restriction nevertheless fulfils the demands. The headings are arranged in a subject index that is unfolded before the testee like a menu. The physician is asked to select a heading, turn up the page and choose an option. Every page reveals a number of options, each of them provided with a code which corresponds to an answer. This answer is read by the experimenter and handed over to the physician. Unforeseen questions were answered ad lib by the experimenter. An accompanying observer notes down the codes, the sequence of answering cards, the time and remarkable elements of professional behaviour. The physician is free to elicit all data appropriate and to advance through the paper patient according to his own choice. There were no time constraints. After the workup, the testee enters the phase of "stimulated recall" on basis of the compiled cards and the observer's notes.

The investigators interviewed sixteen general practitioners and sixteen consulting internists. Each "patient" passed a number of consulting visits sometimes ranging over a couple of months.

Four aspects of working methods were investigated:

- minuteness of medical procedure

- kind of information (psycho-social versus medical)

- uniformity of procedure and conformity within groups

- the role of hypotheses in the hypothetico-deductive strategy

The study underlines the conclusions of Smith and McWhinney (1975). Several problems of simulation can be distinguished in this study such as:

- the cueing effect. The investigators tried to limit this effect in two ways:

(a) Disclosing only parts of the format

(b) Using the hypothesis that large numbers of options diminish the cueing effect. This hypothesis was not tested.

- the options did not cover the whole field. Three hundred and sixty-four questions posed by physicians could not be answered. This incompleteness varied between 5% and 20%.

- within the sequence of consulting visits, the same options (the format did not change) could give rise to different replies.

- a number of questions had to be answered by improvisation.

- the format had to be structured according to the chosen hypothetico-deductive strategy.

Conditions for Paper Patient Models

Can we formulate conditions for models of patient simulations out of these thoughts? Let us consider the function of simulation in teaching, that of learning and measuring clinical competence. Nowadays we are convinced that learning and practising clinical competence is not only gained by experience. The learning of problem-solving and decision-making is one of the most neglected parts in medical education.

To learn these skills it is essential to know the content and structure of the medical process or the various medical processes:

1. The content: the data and symbols which compose together the basis for diagnosis and therapeutic management. Unfortunately, most of these data and symbols are founded on implicit, individual knowledge based on personal experience. As mentioned previously, diagnoses are not devoid of value judgments and differ from physician to physician.

2. The structure: the rules, laws and sequences binding the data to verifiable or refutable concepts of disease or health status of the patient. It is assumed that the problem-solving process of physicians is a hypothetico-deductive one. As far as there is a training in these skills, it is attuned to this one technique. But one has to realise that this technique will be applied in daily practice by only a small proportion of the physicians. Training programmes aimed at the education of problem-solving techniques with the principles of formal logic, (Bayesian) statistics and problem orientated medical records incur a risk of transmitting a way of thinking that hardly exists in practice and is probably quite useless (Gerritsma & Smal, 1982).

So far, simulation models are built on a number of assumptions. We can now formulate a list of wishes, conditions, criteria for a simulation model that meets the demands of education and research.

1. Case histories as obtained from medical records or composed by expert groups must be replaced by storage of a patient's data highly devoid of value judgements.

2. Data acquisition and storage must be uniform and unambiguous.

3. Data storage must not be submitted to a predetermined processing mode.

4. Data must come from as many sources as possible: patient, relatives, physicians, nurses, social workers etc.

5. Data must be gathered by an independent collector from real situations.

6. Data must be stored in the system easily and quickly (a high production rate).

7. The retrieval of the data by the testee/trainee must allow an individual workup through the case.

8. No cueing allowed.

9. Preferably the "paper patient" is addressed by the decision-maker verbally. This implies the interposition of an experimenter between decision-maker and "paper patient".

10. The experimenter must be a trained person acquainted with medical jargon; able to handle a large number of scenarios; and not influence the candidate.

11. The system, including the experimenter, must allow a realistic provision of answers in a given time.

12. The simulation must approximate the setting and time constraints of the day-to-day professional activities of the physician.

13. The scoring must be based on what really happens in general practice.

14. The scoring variables and their weights must be founded on a reliable and verifiable general practitioners's data base.

15. The simulation must meet the aforementioned qualities of validity and reliability.

REFERENCES

Charvat, J., McGuire, C. H., Parsons, V. (1968): A Review of the Nature and Uses of Examinations in Medical Education, W.H.O., Public Health Paper 2.

Cronbach, L. J. Meehl, P. E. (1955): Construct Validity in Psychological Tests, Psychol. Bull., 52, 281-302.

Dombal, F. T. de, Horrocks, J. C., Staniland, J. R., Gill, P. W. (1971): Simulation of Clinical Diagnosis: A Comparative Study, Brit. Med. J., 2, 575-577.

Elstein, A. S., Shulman, L. S., Sprafka, S. A. (1978): Medical Problem-solving, An Analysis of Clinical Reasoning, Cambridge, Harvard University Press

Gerritsma, J. G. M., Smal, J. A. (1982): De Werkwijze van Huisarts en Internist, Utrecht, W. U. Bunge.

Glaser, R., Damrin, D. E., Gardner, F. M. (1952): The Tab Item Technique for the Measurement of Proficiency in Diagnostic Problem-solving Tasks, Champaign, University of Illinois, Bureau of Research and Service.

Groot, A. D. de (1961): Methodologie. Grondslagen van Onderzoek en Denken in de Gedragswetenschappen, 's-Gravenhage, Mouton & Co.

Harless, W. G., Drennon, G. G., Marxer, J. J., Root, J. A., Miller, G.E. Case (1971): A Computer-Aided Simulation of the Clinical Encounter, J. Med. Educ., 46, 443-448.

Helfer, R. E., Slater, C. H. (1971): Measuring the Process of Solving Clinical Diagnostic Problems, Brit. J. Med. Educ., 5, 48--52.

Kagan, N. (1973): Can Technology Help Us toward Reliability in Influencing Human Interaction? Educat. Technology, 13, 44-51.

Kleinmuntz, B. (1963): Profile Analysis Revisited: A Heuristic Approach, J. Couns. Psychol., 10, 315-321.

McCarthy, W. H., Gonella, J. S. (1967): The Simulated Patient Management Problem: A Technique for Evaluating and Teaching Clinical Competence, Brit. J. Med. Educ., 1, 348-352.

McGaghie, W. C. (1980): Medical Problem-Solving; A Re-Analysis, J. Med. Educ., 55, 912-920.

McGuire, C. H. (1976): Simulation Technique in the Teaching and Testing of Problem-solving Skills, J. Res. Sci. Teaching, 13, 89-100.

Pauker, S. G., Gorry, G. A., Kassirer, J. P., Schwartz, W. B. (1976): Towards the Simulation of Clinical Cognition. Taking a Present Illness by Computer, Am. J. Med., 60, 981-996.

Rimoldi, H. J. A. (1961): The Test of Diagnostic Skills, J. Med. Educ., 36, 73-79.

Segers, J. H. G. (1977): Sociologische Onderzoeksmethoden, Assen, Van Gorkum.

Smith, D. H., McWhinney, J. R. (1975): Comparison of the Diagnostic Methods of Family Physicians and Internists, J. Med. Educ., 50, 264-270.

Tamblyn, R., Barrow, H. S. (1978a): Evaluation Trail of the P4 System: Problem Based Learning System, Monograph 4 4/78 McMaster University, Hamilton.

Tamblyn, R., Barrow, H. S. (1978b): Teaching Guide for the P4 System: Problem Based Learning System, Monograph 5 4/78, McMaster University, Hamilton

Taylor T. R. (1972): Computer-Assisted Instruction in Medical Education, Prog. Learn. Educ. Technol., 9/5, 272-283.

Uberla, K. (1980): Methodological Limitations in the Analysis of Medical Activities, Meth. Inf. Med., 19, 7-10.

23
Discussion of the Papers by Bentsen and Ridderikhoff

Paul Keith Hodgkin

In the first of these two papers, Professor Bentsen brings us up to date with the enormous effort that has been made over recent years to try and reduce the chaos of primary care terms used by different individuals and in different countries. His vision of one language common to all workers in the field is an inspiring attempt to reduce the Babel of primary care labels and to clarify what each of them means. Fleshing out of some sections remains to be done and others require full field testing but the broad outlines are now clearly visible and it is an impressive sight.

Several key points surfaced in the discussion. Firstly, the classification of disease itself tends to change how general practitioners view and code the morbidity in front of them. The need for careful and standardised use of terms is at times in conflict with the vague and fluid presentation of incompletely differentiated problems. Two possible solutions to this were discussed:

a) to ensure that GP's did not do their own coding. In this way they are free to use whatever label they feel most appropriate.

b) the use of clustering like diagnoses with like as recently presented by Schneeweiss et al. (1983).

Secondly, the classifications are not intended as a kind of monolithic Esperanto to be applied uniformly everywhere. Local conditions will clearly dictate variations. However, the hierarchical structure of the codes means that with a little care such local versions can be made compatible with the broader classifications.

Thirdly, it should be remembered that these classifications (including ICHPPC-2) represent work in progress rather than the final classification.

Following the presentation of Dr Ridderikhoff's paper on patient simulation, the discussion centred on the need for flexibility in using this technique. The opportunities and difficulties of using simulation for teaching, assessment and research are all quite different and this needs to be borne in mind when deciding which, if any, method is most suitable. It was also apparent that within the UK comparatively little work is currently being done on simulation although it is used quite extensively by some departments as a teaching tool. Interest was expressed in the further development of Dr Ridderikhoff's symptom-based simulations.

REFERENCES

Schneewiess, R., Rosenblatt, D., Cherkin, D., Kirkwood, R., and Hart, G., (1983). Diagnosis clusters: A new tool for analysing the content of ambulatory care. Medical Care, XXI, 1.

24
Overview and Implications for Medical Education

George A. Brown

This paper provides an overview of the earlier papers in this volume and it considers their implications for medical education and in particular for postgraduate education in general practice.

Rather than recite a litany of the findings and discussion points in each paper, I outline an interpretive framework which may help the reader to reflect upon the ideas presented by the other contributors to this volume, their own experiences of doctor-patient consultations and their own clinical thinking. This overview then provides a basis for the discussion of the implications for courses, assessment, learning and teaching in postgraduate education for general practitioners.

OVERVIEW

Research on doctor-patient consultations, including studies of decision-making, is based upon a spectrum of underlying methodologies and models. At one end of the spectrum is the pole of scientific explanation which Giorgi (1976) labelled as erklarung and at the other is personal understanding which is labelled verstehen.

The cluster of values associated with erklarung include the development of covering laws and models which enable explanations and predictions to be made[1]. There is an underlying concern with quantitative measurement, with problems of measuring reliability and validity and with, as far as possible, identical repetition of experiments. Associated with the mode of scientific explanation is often an interest in the organic, in disease-centred models and in the search for mathematically-based generalisations within a closed system of concepts.

---

[1] The generalisation of experience alone may be sufficient for prediction but not for explaining an organic condition.

SCIENTIFIC EXPLANATION	PERSONAL UNDERSTANDING
Experimentation	Plus other forms of research
Quantity	Quality
Measurement	Meaning
Reactions	Intentions
Repetition	Related phenomena
Independent Observer	Participant Observer
Statistical Prediction	"Clinical" Prediction
Statistical generalisation	Generalisations based on cases

Figure 1   Some polar contrasts of research methodology

In contrast, the pole of verstehen is concerned with personal understanding, with meanings rather than measurement, with intentions rather than directly observable actions. From such a standpoint doctor-patient consultations are seen as sets of unique thought-related events, each of which is influenced by a particular cluster of conditions including the doctor's history, the problem and the patient's history. Instead of searching for covering laws, one looks at how an individual induces relevant hypotheses or explanatory principles, how he or she detects regularities and arrives at decisions. Associated with the mode of personal understanding is often an interest in the individual's conceptions of illness, in patient-centred models and in a search for interpretations and meanings within the consultation.

These two poles, erklarung and verstehen are manifest in psychology (Giorgi, 1966; Ricoeur, 1981) in studies of consultations and in the papers presented in this volume[2]. For example, the papers presented by Fox, Ridderikhoff, Bentsen, and Rector and Dodson are more akin to the pole of erklarung than verstehen whereas the papers by Gale and Marsden, Essex and by Brooke and Sheldon using the repertory grid[3] are closer to the pole of verstehen. McWhinney (this publication) discussed various models which manifest the range of models of clinical decision-making.

The tension between the erklarung and verstehen approaches are also manifest within individuals, within the medical curriculum and within programmes of education for general practitioners. However the poles of scientific explanation and of personal understanding provide only a preliminary sort of the papers presented here. Within the spectrum of methodologies available one can identify five models for researching doctor-patient consultations and these models, in varying degrees, are manifest in the papers of this volume.

MODELS OF RESEARCH

A. The Physiological Model

The physiological model is based on the premise that given a set of theoretical statements T and given a set of conditions W an entity X will act in an observable manner Z.

Probabilities may be assigned to Z, but W and Z are relatively independent of X. Thus given a theory of increased fat intake in cholelithiasis will produce flatulent dyspepsia - a bacon and egg breakfast will probably produce discomfort and belching in a patient with hypochondiacal opacities (on straight abdominal X-ray films).

---

[2] The poles of erklarung and verstehen are convenient first approximations. There is, however a deeper concept, that of intuition. This seems to develop through experience of scientific explanation and personal understanding. Thus, for example, when reading scientific papers one can sometimes sense that there is a flaw in the paper or when diagnosing a patient one can sense that one's understanding is inadequate. Neither intuition may, initially, be articulated and until it is it cannot be subjected to test.

[3] The repertory grid is a rogue case. The background theory is akin to personal understanding whereas the grid itself more closely resembles the characteristics of scientific explanation.

The model is basic to physiology, anatomy, to most pre-clinical subjects and to pathology. There are, of course, individual differences and hence the relationship between W and Z is influenced by the particular entity X. The model tries to establish generalisations and to minimise individual differences. It focusses primarily upon signs rather than symptoms, it ignores in large measure the constructions of the patient and it assumes that meanings and the language used by doctors and patients are identical.

This model obviously has value when the problem has been identified as predominantly somatic. It has less value in diagnosis and in patient-management involving salient social or psychological factors.

B. The Information Technology Model

This model in its strongest form is based upon the assumption that human thinking is analogous to computer processes. Thus the use of algorithms, decision trees and error analysis are used to explain how doctors take clinical decisions. The menu-driven model is the most obvious example of this approach. It is assumed that a doctor has a master list, searches through this for the appropriate diagnosis, checks it out and if it is not appropriate returns to the master list.

In its weaker form the information technology model assumes that a support system of information retrieval and its extended memory will enable the doctor to make more accurate diagnoses and management plans.

This model is implicit in the work reported here by Fox, Rector and Dodson, Taylor, and Dunwoodie.

The model assumes that language and meanings of doctors and patients are, if not identical, then congruent.

C. The Epidemiological Model

This model is concerned with describing the range of factors which influence the doctor-patient consultation. It uses statistics to summarise trends, to make tentative generalisations and to predict likely outcomes. As such it provides a broad canvas of the factors at work. Unlike the physiological model, repeat measures in this model are used to estimate change rather than to test validity. The model draws on reports, which may be structured or unstructured, or individual respondents rather than upon direct observation. The users of the model do not usually claim to be able to predict accurately the process or product of a doctor-patient consultation. The work of Cartwright (1967, 1981) and more recently of Brooke and Sheldon (this volume) exemplifies this approach.

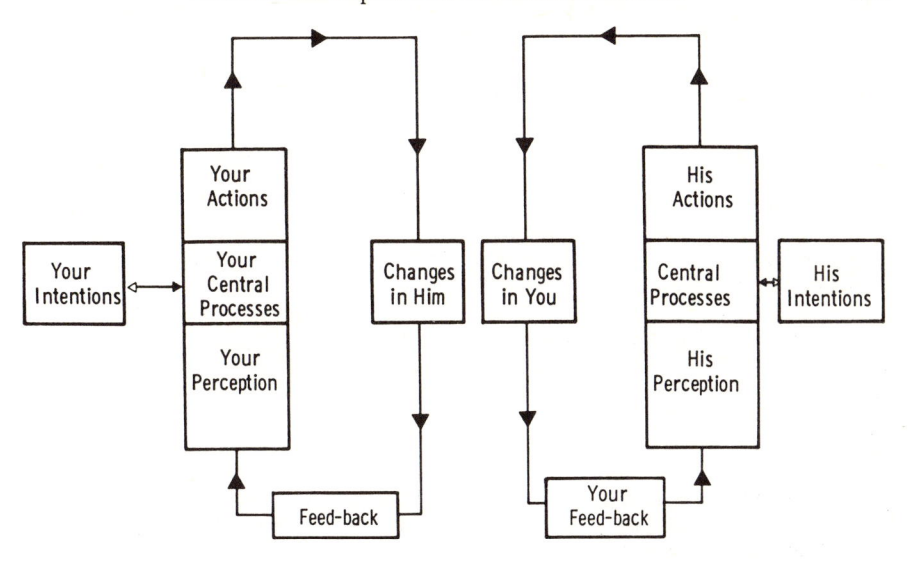

FIG. 2

D. The Social Skills Model

This model is based upon the work of Argyle (1970, 1981).

In its truncated form (A) it indicates that a doctor may have certain intentions which activate central processes containing knowledge, attitudes, values and skills of diagnosis and management. This activation leads to actions including questioning, explaining, listening, observing, which in turn produce long or short term observable changes in the patient. The short term changes are perceived, and interpreted. These interpretations may modify the doctor's specific intentions or they may confirm them.

This truncated model is at the heart of many training programmes in doctor-patient consultations (Pendleton et al, 1984). It is concerned primarily with helping a doctor to analyse and understand his/her actions and with providing opportunities to refresh and refine the skills of diagnosis and management. In so doing it may also provide information on common strengths and weaknesses (see, Stott, this publication, and Maguire, 1981) and on difficulties in communication (Pendleton et al, 1983).

It may suggest guidelines for action. However, the model is not primarily concerned with prediction and control although some users of the model may, unwittingly, wish to impose a robotic approach to training.

The extended version of the model takes into account the patient's intentions, central processes, actions, and perceptions of the doctor.

In so doing it provides an initial model for exploring and understanding patients as persons with their own intentions, perceptions and interpretations.

E. The Hermeneutic Model

Hermeneutics was originally the study of texts and their meanings (Ricoeur, 1981). In more recent years it has become the study of intentions and meanings for the participants in social situations. Thus the doctor-patient consultation may be viewed as a text analogue and techniques of analysing verbal and body language applied to tease out the intentions of doctors and patients, the meanings they attach to various words and sentences and how they construct their notions of various diseases, of illness, health and, more fundamentally, of themselves.

Hermeneutics is in part based upon two concepts of Greek origin, the noetic and noematic. The noetic refers to that level and depth of feeling and thought which is unknowable. The noematic refers to the level of feelings, thoughts which may be articulated with varying degrees of sophistication. The noematic is expressed in language which is, to some extent, idiosyncratic. Doctors interpret noematic in their own personal languages and they recreate the noematic of their patients in terms of their own noematic which may resonate with their own noetic[4]. In this way, according to the hermeneuticists, we develop our personal understanding of others and their condition. The model is deep and for those with a predilection for physiological models it may seem unnecessarily complex. However, it does remind us forcefully that our interpretations of a patient are based upon not just signs and symptoms but upon signs and upon symptoms that have first been construed by the patient, then articulated by the patient and then construed and interpreted by us.

Hermeneutics makes no claims to produce covering laws nor does it seek to predict and still less to control. It does however stress that personal understanding may be deepened by reflecting upon our experiences, on how we construe, interpret and think and that in so doing we may develop and test the intuitions, prototypes and private theories which have sedimented in our semantic and episodic memories.

This process of matching and interpreting present experience against past experience sets up a dissonance which is resolved either by rejecting the validity of the present experience, assimilating the experience into one's existing cognitive structures, or by accommodating the experience - thereby changing the cognitive structures[5]. In a profound sense the model implies that doctors are their own researchers[6].

---

[4] This metaphorical description is probably the kernel of how intuition operates (see previous note).

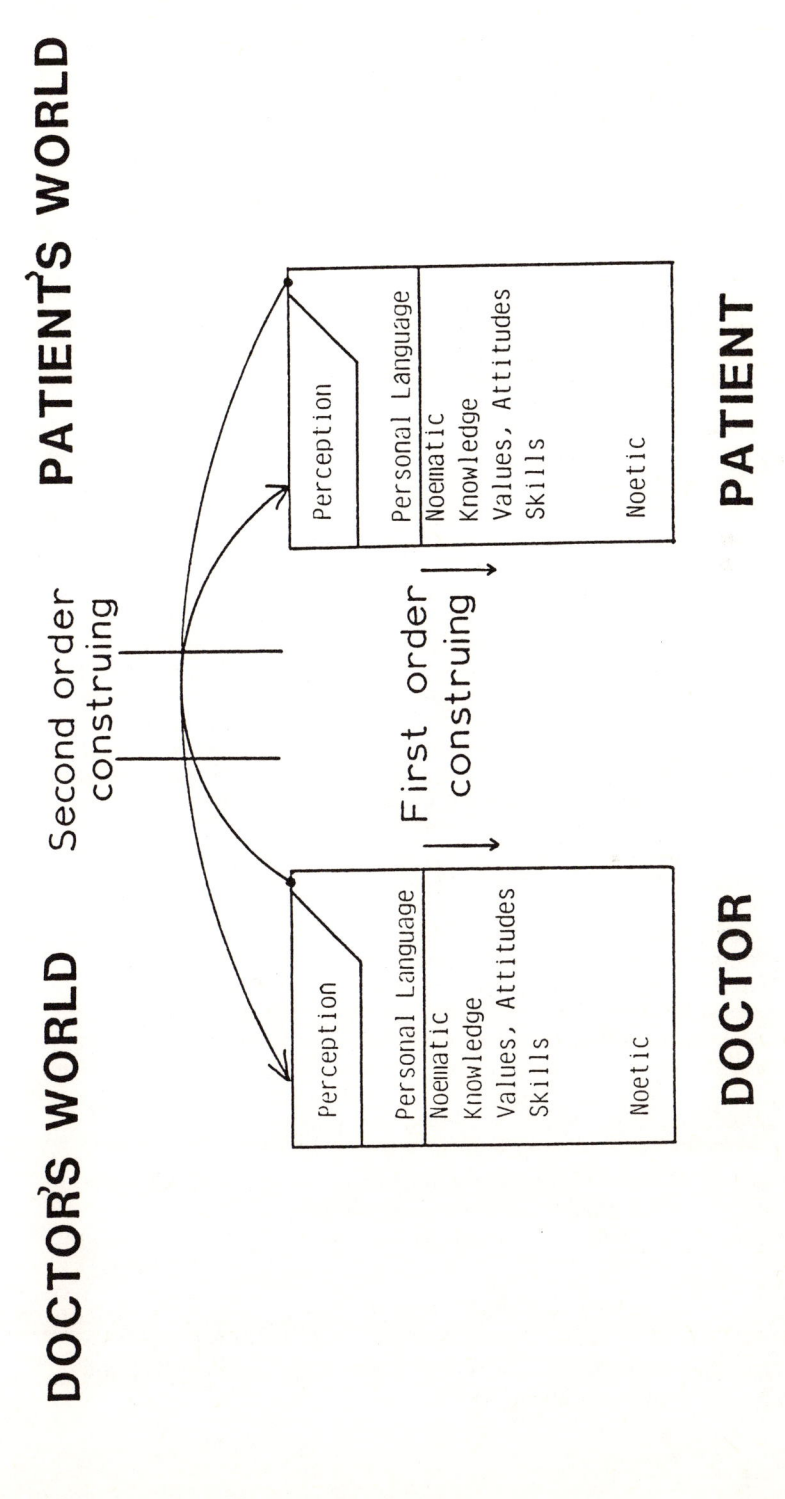

Overview and Implications for Medical Education 263

PATIENT'S WORLD

PATIENT

DOCTOR'S WORLD

DOCTOR

Second order construing

First order construing

Perception | Personal Language | Noematic Knowledge | Values, Attitudes | Skills | Noetic

Perception | Personal Language | Noematic Knowledge | Values, Attitudes | Skills | Noetic

FIG. 3

The model is explicit in the clinical study of depressives by Rowe (1978) in which she concludes that prediction of individuals was impossibly complex and that the most she could do was "to recognise the change and so behave in what I (she) hoped was an appropriate way". The model provides an extended rationale for the seminal work of Balint (1957) and a rationale for the work of Byrne and Long (1976). It is implicit in the work of Gale and Marsden on different forms of clinical thinking (this volume) and it is germane to the studies by Essex and Levenstein (this volume).

IMPLICATIONS FOR MEDICAL EDUCATION

Each of the papers in this volume has implications for medical education. When taken together within the interpretive framework provided in the first part of this paper, these implications are even more powerful.

The Medical Curriculum

The medical curriculum is shot through with the notions of erklarung and verstehen. Scientific approaches predominate in pre-clinical courses, they are stressed in clinical courses and in postgraduate examinations. Yet the practice of medicine depends in large measure upon personal understanding. The assumption underlying most medical curricula is that scientific studies should precede the development of personal understanding. The curriculum experiments at McMaster and Newcastle (1983) are based upon the notion of developing personal understanding and scientific explanations concurrently. The evidence of consecutive and concurrent approaches is not yet available. My suspicion is that other curricular imperatives such as subject territory will prove to be more influential than the global issue of consecutive or concurrent approaches. Rather than tackle the medical curriculum as an entity it may be more appropriate to stress the ability to provide scientific explanation and to develop personal understanding within each subject. In short, I am advocating that more emphasis be placed in assessment and teaching upon thinking and rather less upon knowledge per se (Marton, 1975; Entwistle, 1981; Brown, 1983).

---

[5] The notion of assimilation and accommodation are derived from Piagetian theory (Piaget and Inhalder, 1969). Matching and interpreting seem to me to apply equally to scientific explanation and personal understanding.

[6] Just as professional researchers vary in their capacity to formulate hypotheses and test them so too do practitioners. Both groups develop their research skills by reflecting upon their uses of them and their implicit models of behaviour.

Postgraduate Education for General Practitioners

The above remarks apply to the membership (M.R.C.G.P.) examinations which are predominantly concerned with recall of scientific explanations, to various curricula being devised for trainees and to courses for general practitioners. Clearly courses which provide recent research findings and procedures in clinical subjects are necessary. So too are courses which provide opportunities to refresh and refine one's skills of diagnosis and management and develop one's understanding of patients. Even more important are courses which enable practitioners to integrate within their cognitive frameworks new knowledge, skills and insights of clinical conditions, of patients and of support systems so that they can apply them in their practice and reflect upon their uses.

The General Practitioner as Personal Researcher

Given that the goal of continuing education for all medical practitioners, including general practitioners, is improving patient care, it is appropriate to suggest that every doctor should be a researcher. By this I do not mean that medical practitioners should be involved in drug trials, epidemiological surveys and other large scale researches. I do mean that every doctor should be his/her own researcher who incorporates relevant scientific knowledge and understanding of patients into his repertoire.

The models of how research is conducted on doctor-patient consultations and the strengths and weaknesses of those models, all have relevance to the task of the doctor as personal researcher. It may be argued that courses should be designed and implemented which introduce and explore these models in depth so that the participants are not only aware of the models, their power and limitations, but are also aware of why they prefer some models to others. Clearly predilection for a particular model is a function of personality values and orientations to knowledge. By studying the various models and one's preferences, one will be deepening one's understanding of how one learns as well as deepening understanding of doctor-patient consultations - and through knowing how one learns, one improves one's capacity to learn.

Towards a cognitive audit model

So far it has been suggested that all the models for exploring doctor-patient consultations are relevant to the doctor's task and, given that continuing education is to improve patient care, that every doctor should be his/her own researcher. The key to this form of research is reflection upon one's own experience and this is at the heart of the cognitive audit model to which I now turn.

Most general practitioners are familiar with the notion of auditing. Recent advances in the use of computers in general practice can augment and facilitate medical audits (Pringle & Lloyd, 1985) and these techniques could well be introduced into courses during the next few years.

In addition, and perhaps more important, are internal audits of how one thinks, diagnoses, manages, interacts and takes into account patients' perceptions and value systems. This form of audit focusses upon the cognitive processes involved, in scientific knowledge and personal understanding in doctor-patient consultation and, more fundamentally, how we learn. Such reflective learning may be conducted in the privacy of one's study or surgery, but it is likely to be enhanced if it is also conducted in courses. For to learn how one thinks requires strategies and guidelines, opportunities to compare and contrast one's mode of thinking with those of others and opportunities to incorporate new knowledge and skills into one's repertoire.

Teaching Methods in General Practice

Teaching in general practice takes place in courses and in tutorials between trainers and trainees. The courses consist largely of lectures followed by discussion. The lectures may be given by visiting consultants or course organisers who may or may not take into account the relevance of their presentation to general practitioners. The discussions often consist of questions and answers interspersed with brief speeches or observations.

Whilst lectures are an efficient mode of conveying information, they provide no guarantee that the information provided will be incorporated into the listener's active repertoire. This is not to decry all lectures but it is to point out the limitations of lectures as learning devices (Brown, 1978; Brown and Tomlinson, 1980). Similar remarks apply to question-answer sessions. The motives for asking questions of lecturers are mixed but even if the motive is a clarification of the lecturer's viewpoint, the process of learning is limited. Furthermore the cycle of lecture-discussion runs the risk of establishing sub networks of learning which are activated primarily on courses rather than in consultations.

Some courses do use video or audio techniques to help practitioners and trainees to refine and refresh their management skills. Such courses are an active form of learning but there are two common pitfalls. The first is that the video playback is viewed passively. It is not enough to look at doctor-patient consultations, one should look into doctor-patient consultations. To do this one may need guidelines and checklists (Brown, 1984). The second pitfall is that trainers or other members of the group are hasty, even destructive, in their criticisms. Consequently the situation is threatening and learning is blocked.

Both types of courses could be improved by using teaching methods based upon the notions of the cognitive audit model. Human beings probably learn best when they are active, the content is relevant to their experience, they feel safe, the objectives are clearly specified and their needs are satisfied. Hence courses designed to help doctors improve their patient care should be built around activities designed to promote reflection, analysis and thinking. Lectures and discussions should be brief and built around these activities.

Tutorials in the surgery are supposedly an important feature of courses for trainees. My observations of such tutorials are that they are usually mini lectures or disguised vivas. Neither approach is likely to promote learning. If the purpose of tutorials is to develop personal understanding and scientific explanation, then rather more attention needs to be devoted to appropriate tutorial methods based on reflective learning. Indeed the problem of trainer-trainee tutorials is that such apprenticeship is seen as a process of modelling the clinical master rather than mastering the diversity of clinical and research models that are available.

Teaching the teachers of general practice

The rich diversity of findings and models of studying the consultation in this volume are relevant to the work of lecturers, course organisers and trainers in general practice. If these findings and methods are to be incorporated into their teaching repertoire then methods of teaching have to be used which stimulate active use of the findings and models. The problem of teaching teachers of general practice is therfore isomorphic with the problem of teaching trainees and general practitioners. It follows that the appropriate methods of teaching are those which provide opportunities for reflection, analysis and thinking about teaching the scientific and personal aspects of the consultations. The methods of teaching experienced would then be consonant with the methods which they would be using on their courses and in their surgeries.

SUMMARY

This paper has outlined briefly the models which underpin research in general practice and the doctor-patient consultation in particular. These models may be set upon a continuum which has at one pole the notions of scientific explanation, prediction and control, and at the other, the notion of personal understanding and the search for meaning. It has been argued that all of these models are relevant to the work of general practitioners and that to improve patient care it is necessary for practitioners to become their own researchers. For this to be achieved courses and teaching methods have to be developed which are based upon systematic reflection, analysis and thinking of the processes involved in the consultation and in learning. Physician know thyself, thy patients and their problems.

REFERENCES

Argyle, M., (1970). Social Interaction. Methuen, London.

Argyle, M., (ed) (1981). Social Skills and Health. Methuen, London.

Balint, M., (1957). The Doctor, his Patient and the Illness. Pitman Medical Publishing, London.

Brown, G.A., (1978). Lecturing and Explaining. London: Methuen.

Brown, G.A., (1983). Styles of Learning: Implications for medical teaching. Medical Teacher, 5, 2, 52-56.

Brown, G.A., (1984). Analysing Doctor-patient Interactions. Nottingham: mimeo.

Brown, G.A., and Tomlinson, D.M., (1980). How to Improve Lecturing. Medical Teacher, 1, 3, 128-135.

Byrne, P.S., and Long, B.E., (1976). Doctors Talking to Patients. HMSO, London.

Cartwright, A., (1967). Patients and their Doctors. Routledge, Kegan and Paul, London.

Cartwright, A., (1981). General Practice Revisited. Routledge, Kegan and Paul, London.

Entwistle, N., (1981). Styles of Learning. Wiley, Chichester.

Giorgi, A., (1965, 1966). Phenomenology and Experimental Psychology. Review of Existential Psychology and Psychology, 5, 228-238; 6, 37-50.

Giorgi, A., (1976). Phenomenology and the Foundation of Psychology. In Nebraska Symposium on Motivation. (ed. J.K. Cole). University of Nebraska Press, Lincoln.

Maguire, P., (1981). Doctor Patient Skills. In: Social Skills and Health. (ed. M. Argyle). Metheun, London.

Marton, F., (1975). In: How Students Learn. (eds. N. Entwistle and D. Hounsell). University of Lancaster, Lancaster.

McWhinney, I.R., (1985) Patient-Centred and Doctor-Centred Models of Clinical Decision-Making. This volume.

Pendleton, D.A., Brouwer, H., and Jaspars, J. (1983) Journal of Language and Social Psychology, 2, 17-36.

Pendleton, D.A., Schofield, J., Toto, P., and Havelock, P. (1984) The Consultation. Oxford: Oxford University Press.

Newcastle, (1983). Collected papers on Medical Education. University of Newcastle, New South Wales.

Pendleton, D.A., Schofield, T.P.C., Tate, P.K., and Havelock, P.B., (1983). The Consultation: an Approach to Teaching and Learning. Oxford University Press, Oxford.

Piaget, J., and Inhalder, B. (1969). The Psychology of the Child. Routledge, Kegan and Paul, London.

Pringle, M. and Lloyd, R., (1985). Uses of Computers in General Practice. Oxford University Press, London. (in press).

Ricoeur, P., (1978). The Role of Metaphor. London: Routledge, Kegan and Paul, London.

Ricoeur, P., (1981). Hermeneutics and the Human Sciences. Cambridge University Press, Cambridge.

Rowe, D., (1978). The Experience of Depression. Wiley, Chichester.

Stott, N.C.H., (1985) The Surface Anatomy of Primary Health Care - Does Consultation Analysis Contribute? This volume.